General Surgery, Anesthesiology and Diagnostic Imaging

General Surgery, Anesthesiology and Diagnostic Imaging

Authors :

Dr. RAMESH RATHOD
M. V. Sc (Surg & Rad), Ph.D, PGDCR, PGDMLS.
Veterinary Officer
Department of Animal Husbandry and Veterinary Services
Bagalkot, Karnataka

Dr. L. RANGANATH
M. V. Sc (Surg & Rad), Ph.D, FISVS, FISACP
Professor and Head
Department of Veterinary Surgery and Radiology
Veterinary College, Hebbal, Bangalore, Karnataka

Dr. M. S. VASANTH
M. V. Sc (Surg & Rad), Ph.D, FISVS, FISACP
Dean
Veterinary College, Hassan, Karnataka

Dr. B. N. NAGARAJU
M. V. Sc (Surg & Rad), Ph.D, FISVS
Professor
Department of Veterinary Surgery and Radiology
Veterinary College, Hebbal, Bangalore, Karnataka

SSPH

SATISH SERIAL PUBLISHING HOUSE
403, Express Tower, Commercial Complex
Azadpur, Delhi-110033 (India)
Phone : 011-27672852, Fax : 91-11-27672046
e-mail : info@satishserial.com, hkjain1975@yahoo.com
Website : www.satishserial.com

Published by :

SATISH SERIAL PUBLISHING HOUSE

403, Express Tower, Commercial Complex, Azadpur, Delhi-110033 (INDIA)
Phone : 011-27672852 Fax : 91-11-27672046
E-mail : info@satishserial.com, hkjain1975@yahoo.com

ISBN 978-93-85055-82-9

Composed, Designed & Printed in India

This Book is Dedicated to
Veterinary Profession

Preface

The book General Surgery, Anesthesiology and Diagnostic Imaging is written exclusively for Undergraduate Veterinary Students. In order to have complete information concerned to Veterinary Council of India syllabus in one text, this book is framed. From the view of the students as there will be short duration to Collect complete information during the semester, the students can't get everything in a single text, with that intention, the present book is prepared.

During the last decade there have been tremendous advances in non-invasive imaging technologies. Now-a-days it is possible to scan an entire patient by CT and MRI with high spatial resolution and with exquisite tissue contrast within seconds or minutes. Contrast agents can be applied and their accumulation monitored dynamically to gain functional data about tissue vascularisation, perfusion and permeability. In addition, imaging modalities that are highly sensitive to administered radiolabelled probes like PET and SPECT are more focused in this text along with figures.

I request the students to refer other text books, where still extra information is needed as it is very difficult to cover each and everything in a single text. Minor errors are unavoidable so I request the readers kindly to bring it to our notice so that we will correct it while printing the next issues. We hope that the information provided in the text will help in gaining the knowledge to the readers concerned to Surgery, Anesthesiology and Diagnostic Imaging.

I thank God for my profession and the opportunity to accrue the information and knowledge that I feel are most pertinent for veterinary students and guide practitioners, many of whom I have been fortunate to interact. We are thankful to Karnataka, Veterinary, Animal and Fisheries Sciences, University located at Bidar and Department of Surgery and Radiology for providing the platform in publishing this book. Lastly your valuable suggestions for improving the quality of the book in future are awaited.

Thank you

Authors

Contents

GENERAL SURGERY

1

Introduction

Surgery is a branch of Veterinary science or medical science which deals with the treatment of the disease or wound or injury using operation or surgical procedure. The term surgery is derived from Greek word chirurgia (Cheiron-hand, ergon- work i.e. work with hand).

Development of Surgery

Veterinary Surgery is as old as civilization. In India, Veterinary practice goes to 1800 BC, patients consisted of Horses, Elephants and Cattle Simultaneously Similar practices were carried in Egypt and Greece.

In Greek period HIPPOCRATES (460-310) an important development in human medicine began at that time veterinary medicine was also in parallel with human medicine.

Greek man stretch recalls treatment of rabies by resection of Lyssa which means cutting sublingual fold and they believed that to be a worm which causes Rabies.

Romans added little for advancement of distending disease of dog and cat they believed that tail docking method of prophylaxis for rabies.

Spaying in bitches was practiced as early as 1576 by Flank. Spay-devoid of ovaries.

- Progress was slow till 18th century. In 18th century surgery was considered as a trade and not a profession.

- 1760 Claude Bernard, started first Veterinary school in Lyon of France, this was established to study certain disease of domestic animals.
- 19th century, an era of scientific achievement began.
- Mortein in 1846, Publicity and demonstration of ether anesthesia in Baster city Masachusstes for tooth extraction (fig.1).
- Louis Pasture and Joseph Lister 1897 – 1912 evolutional surgery by following Asepsis & Antisepsis (fig.2).
- Pean popularized use of forceps to control haemorrhages.
- Halsted propagated use of rubber gloves during surgery (fig.3).
- Van burgain introduced sterilization by boiling.
- Roentgen introduced X-rays for diagnosis in 1895 (fig. 4). In veterinary practice, Richard Eberlin of Germany is considered to be the "Father of Radiology".

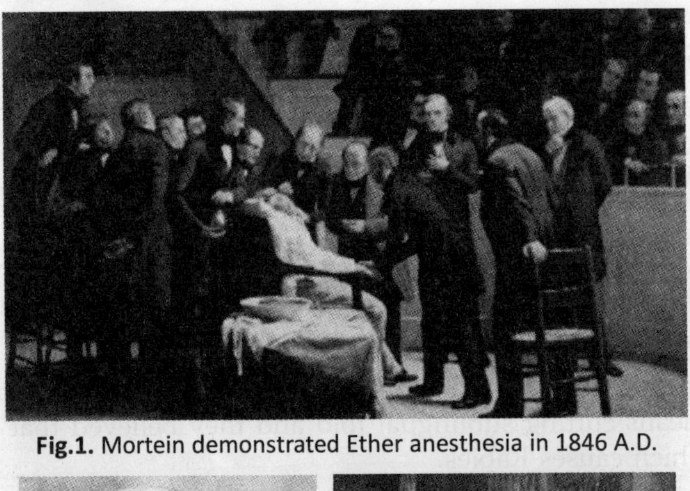

Fig.1. Mortein demonstrated Ether anesthesia in 1846 A.D.

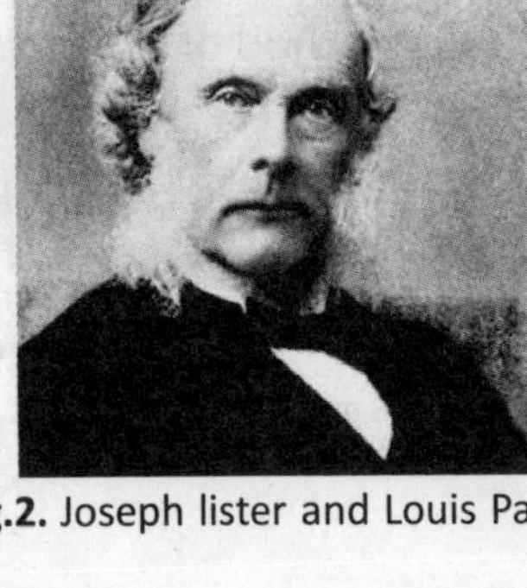

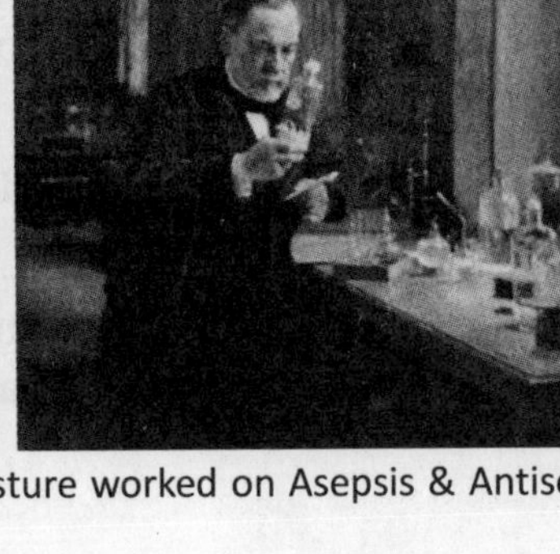

Fig.2. Joseph lister and Louis Pasture worked on Asepsis & Antisepsis

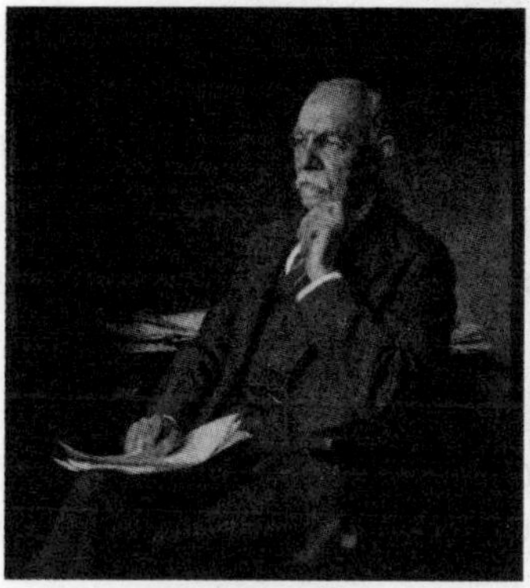

Fig.3. Halsted propagated use of Rubber gloves during surgery

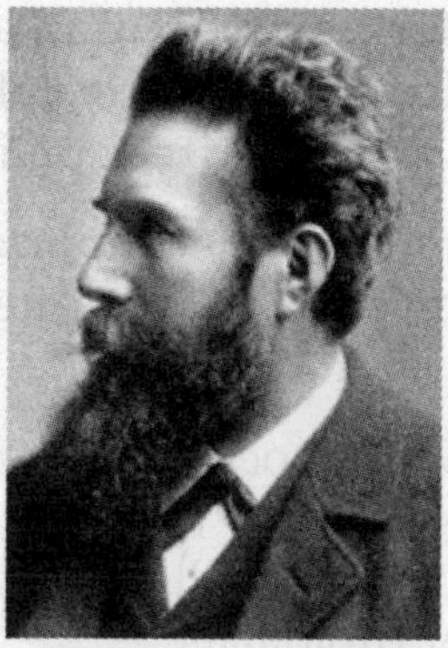

Fig. 4. 1895 A.D- Roentgen Discovered x-rays

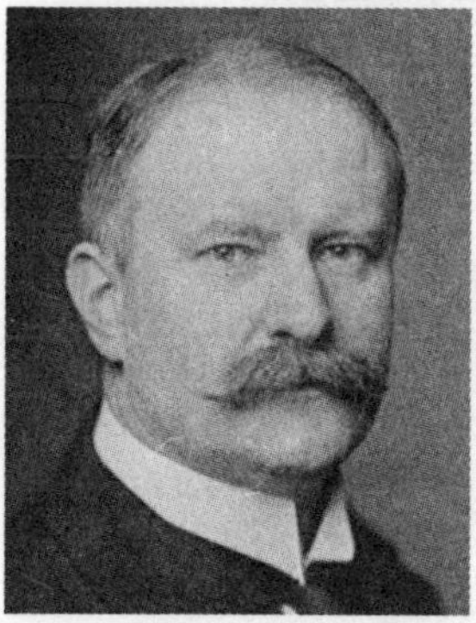

Fig. 5. Bier introduced spinal anesthesia & IVRA (Intravenous Regional Anesthesia)

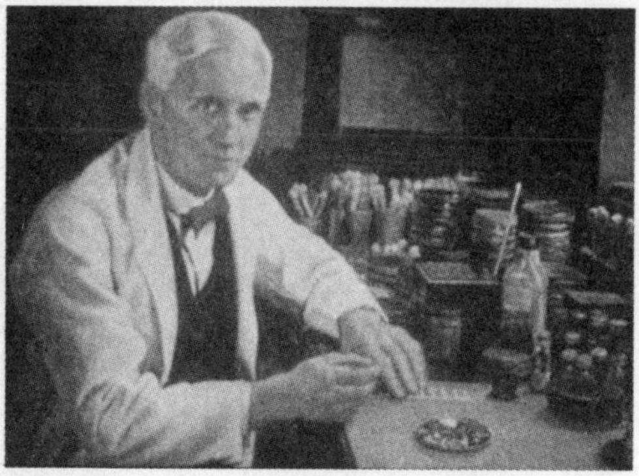

Fig. 6. Alexander Fleming discovered Penicillin

- In 1898 Bier produced spinal anesthesia in animal & also popularized use of IVRA (Intravenous Regional Anesthesia) or Retrograde anesthesia & also Bier's hyperemia technique cranial to the wound by applying an elastic band to compress blood vessels to create passive venous congestion. (fig.5)
- In 20th century lot of development began. Invention of penicillin by Alexander Fleming in 1929 revolutionized more success of surgical procedure with more surgical safety. (fig.6)
- In 20th century development of Barbiturate in 1920-30 made way for safe anesthesia. In veterinary surgery i/v anesthesia is introduced since 1940.
- Schroder in 1933 started orthopaedic surgery in dog.

- Markowits of Canada propagated surgical application of physiological principles like Asepsis in veterinary practices. He also popularized application of Anatomy & physiology in surgery.
- Some of the important veterinarians of 20th century James Archuval, Markourites, Schroder, Frank, Hobdae, Smith, Guard & Lwttal.
- 1965 Association of American College of Veterinary Surgery was established which is a forum for surgical programme. In 1974 American college of veterinary surgery began conducting exams for diplomats.
- 1977 Indian Society of Veterinary Surgery began (ISVS), followed by journal - Indian Journal of Veterinary Surgery.

□□□

2

Classification and Surgical Terminology

Surgery is a branch of medicine which deals with treatment of Diseases & injuries by a manual procedure hands which is synonymous to the CHIRIGUIA.

Chir and "working with hands"

Guia means work

Veterinary surgery is a branch practiced in animals

Aseptic Surgery: Surgery performed with all sterile precautions (using sterile instrument & sterile maneuvers). (fig.7)

Clinical Surgery: Surgery being performed with prefixed date, time Ex: Tumour, Hernia, castration, haematoma. (fig.8)

Emergency Surgery: It is a surgery performed immediately to save the life of a person. Ex: Accident wound, caesarean etc.

Exploratory Surgery: It is performed to arrive at a correct diagnosis & at the same time surgical corrections Ex: Intestinal obstruction, intussusceptions, Rumenotomy, Ceacal dilatation (fig.9)

Reconstructive Surgery: It is performed for correction of deformities & malformation. Ex: Hare lip, cleft palate, contracted tendon. (fig.10)

Plastic Surgery: it is a repair of deformities/ defects either by direct union of parts /transfer of tissue from one part to other area of the body. Ex: peripheral surgery – skin graft – least hair & least sebaceous gland.

Graft: Live tissue transferred from one part to other part from same patient or from a donor. Ex: Kidney, skin damage etc. (fig.11)

Prosthetic: Inanimate thing made from metal, porcelain - denture, hip replacement, knee replacement. (fig.12)

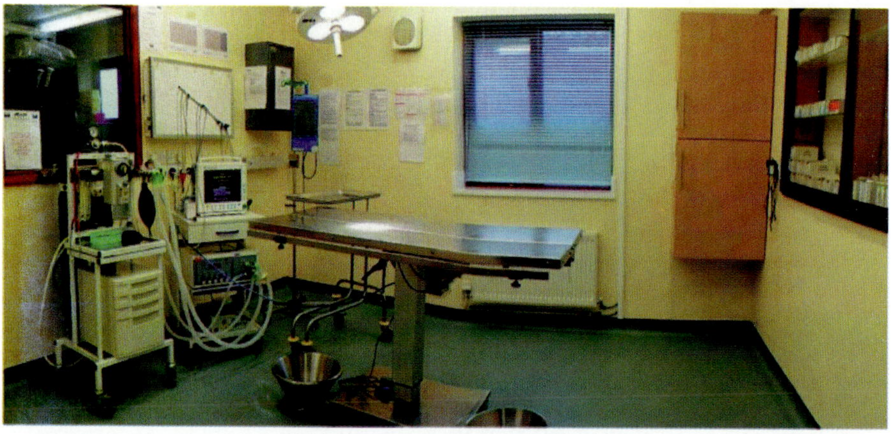

Fig.7. Aseptic operation theatre

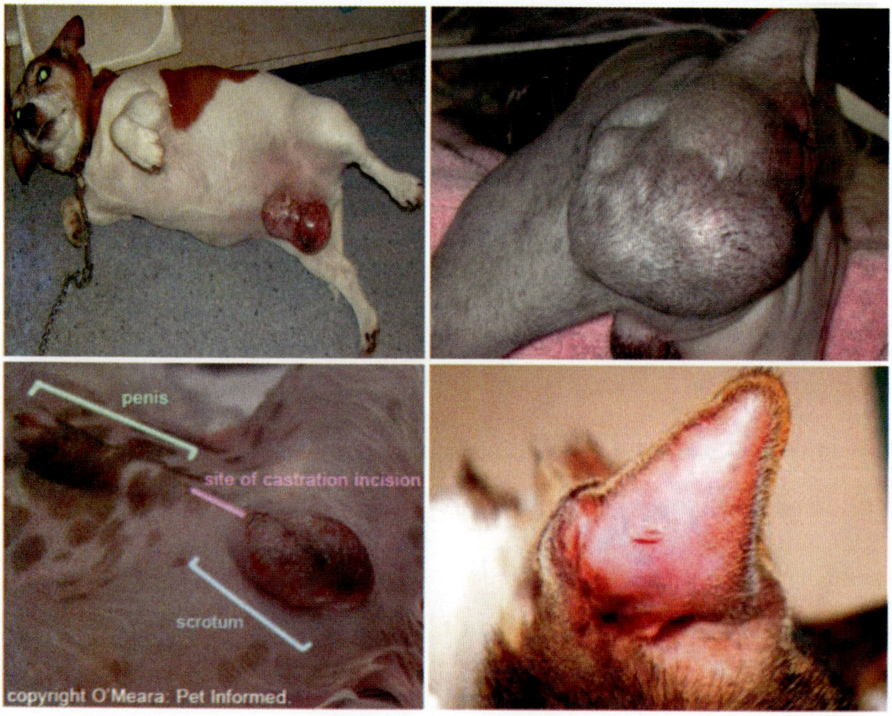

Fig. 8. Clinical Surgeries

(1) Tumor (2) Perineal Hernia (3) Castration (4) Aural Hematoma

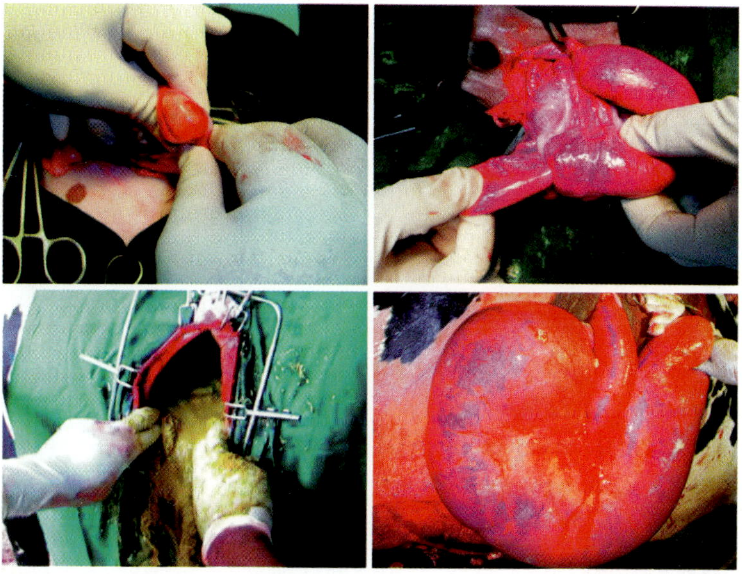

Fig. 9. Exploratory emergency Surgeries (1) Intestinal Obstruction (2) Intussusception (3) Rumenotomy (4) Ceacal Dilation.

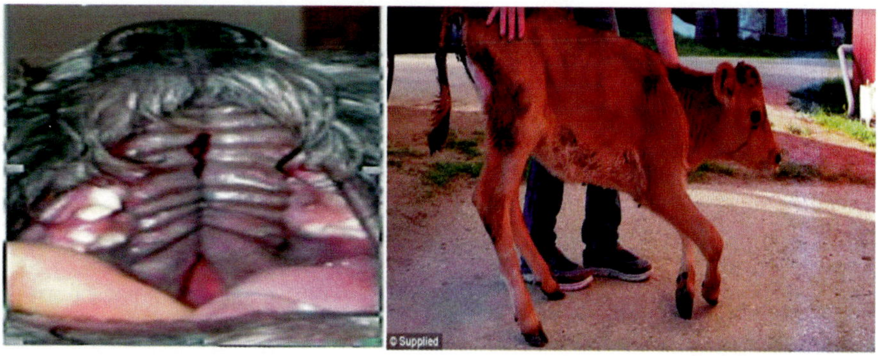

Fig.10. Reconstructive Surgeries (1) Cleft Palate (2) Contracted Tendon

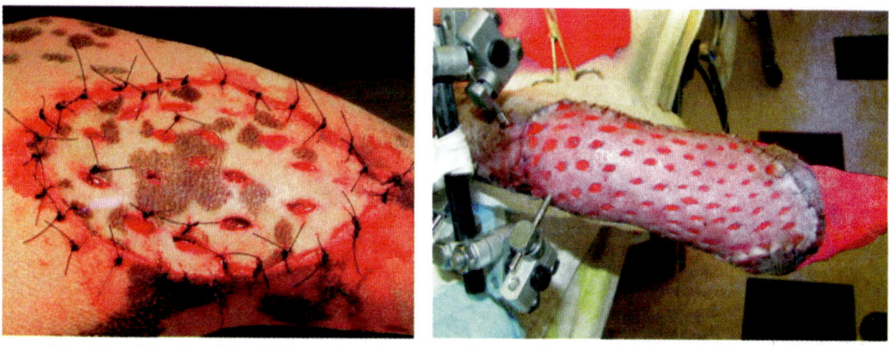

Fig.11. skin Grafting (Live tissue is transferred from one part to other part)

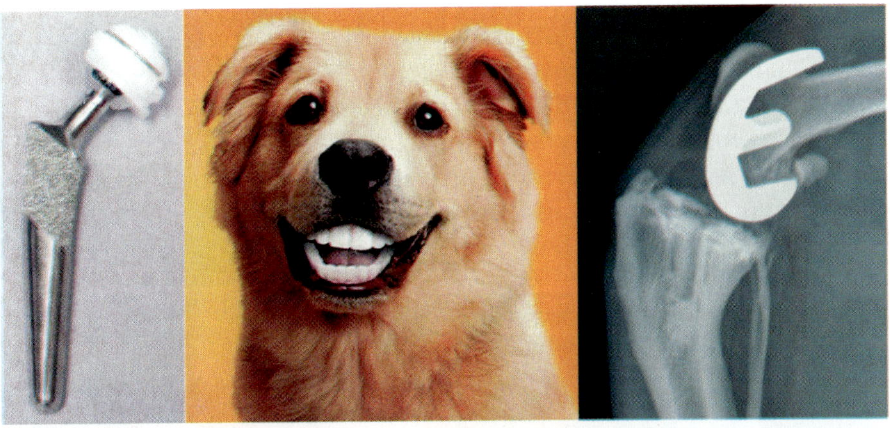

Fig.12. Prosthetics (1) Hip Replacement (2) Porcelain – Denture (3) Knee Replacement

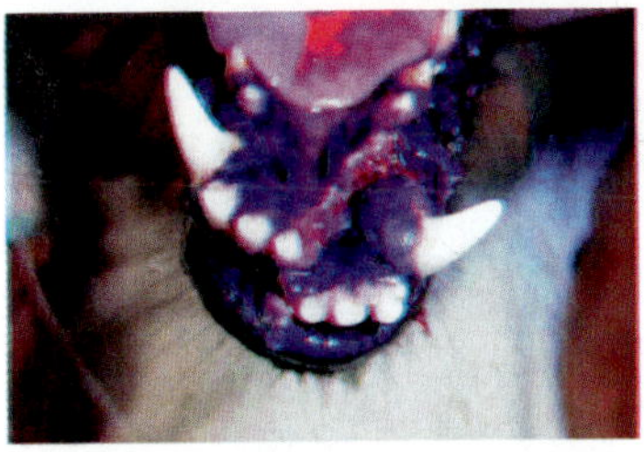

Fig.13. Constructive Surgery (Mandibular Fracture)

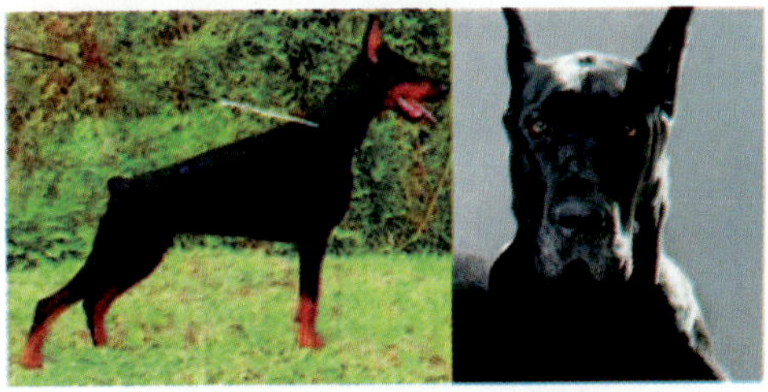

Fig.14. Cosmetic surgery (1) Docking (2) Ear trimming

Constructive Surgery: performed to preserve/restore any desirable part rather than its removal (every attempt is made to conserve the part). Ex: Mandibular Fracture. (fig.13)

Radical Surgery: it is a surgery performed to remove root cause/ source of a disease. Ex: Neoplasm's

Radical Mastectomy - mammary tumour - breast & pectoral muscle & axillary LN.

Radical - leaving no source of disease to continue (Hernia protrusion of visceral organ below the skin)

Cosmetic surgery: it is performed to improve appearance of an Animal. Ex: Docking, Ear trimming. (fig.14)

Experimental Surgery: it is performed to mocking the systematic approach/investigation for academic purpose.

Minor Surgery: Surgical procedure involving no life risk. Ex: castration.

Major Surgery: Most protract time consuming surgery which involves life risk to the patient. Ex: Abdominal Surgery - Spaying.

Urology - Surgery of Urinary system.

Remedial / curative treatment: treatment which cure the disease

Palliative treatment: Treatment given not to cure the disease but to give some relief to the patient ex: cancer - nerve block, Analgesics

Symptomatic treatment: It is a suppressive treatment for symptoms.

Ex: Gastritis - Antacid & anathematic.

1. History Collections/anamnesis - collection of history
   a. Present history
   b. Past history
2. Observation of symptoms:
   a. subjective symptoms - signs
   b. objective symptoms - abnormalities
3. Systematic investigation, palpation, inspection, percussion - (instrument used is plexors) - bloats tympanic sound. Auscultation: Stethoscope–Audible sound produced by heart, GIT.
4. Diagnosis: (a) Tentative diagnosis (b) Final (c) Differential diagnosis-here same symptoms are commonly seen in several diseases.

   Haematemesis - neoplasm, poisoning & renal failure.

   Melenic faeces - parasitic/renal failure.

Reasons for Surgery

1. To save life of the patient
2. To prolong the life of patient
3. To hasten recovery from injury & fracture
4. To make a definitive diagnosis of a disease process
5. To correct deformities / malformation
6. For replacement of any part of the body.

Tenets of Surgery: By Halsted

1. Gentle handling of the Tissues (Syncope)
2. Aseptic surgery
3. Careful Anatomical dissection
4. Control of Haemorrhage (haemostasis)
5. Avoiding dead space – seroma accumulation
6. Minimum number of sutures
7. Immobilization
8. Avoiding suture tension.

□□□

3

General Considerations

Pre-operative consideration

This is to access prognosis of surgery.

1. Nature of surgery
   a. Minor surgery - Local anesthesia ex: Abscess lancing/nail trimming
   b. Major surgery - General Surgery
2. Ability of the patient to withstand surgery & anesthesia we have to assess animal condition, complete history & diagnosis. An anemic patient if subjected to surgery because of low Hb & blood cells count it affect depth of anesthesia.

   Ex: Thiopentone – for anemic patient & for normal patient dosage varies.

   Toxemic patient cannot tolerate anesthesia for this complete information is required:
   a. History of the animal
   b. Hematology
   c. ECG
   d. Temperature-subnormal (temp is not ideal)
   e. Auscultation
3. Assess post operative management & economics required for the surgery.
4. Availability of facilitates & qualified skilled surgeon.

Fixing the time of surgery

Surgery is divided into 2 types:

a. Elective Surgery-fixed according to availability of surgical time.

b. Emergency Surgery - performed at any time of the day.

Elective Surgery is performed

Preferably in early morning there will be time for observation and monitoring the animal. It is easy to prepare the animal by fasting.

There are some of laborious and protracted surgeries, so post operative observation are required.

Preoperative Preparation

Surgical patient selection and preparation require attention to number of details such as, owner counseling, preparation of the animal, preparation of Operation Theater, preparation of surgeon and surgical team. The patient should always receive a complete physical examination, followed by appropriate laboratory backup. A thorough history helps to determine the extent of physical and laboratory examinations. Preoperative information's also allows the comparison of animal's status before and after surgery.

When a surgery is to be performed for relief of disease, considerable care must be exercised in assessing the risks, which the particular animal carries in relation to the anesthetic procedure and surgery. Broadly pre-operative preparations are made and are discussed under following headings.

1. Preparation of surgical instruments and equipments

- The basic knowledge of the material used in the operating room, such as apparel, instruments, sutures and drapes, is essential if one is to master the technique of good aseptic surgical procedure.
- A well-trained surgeon should be familiar with the materials and equipments available, their usefulness, and the methods used in preparing them for surgery.
- All these things play an important role in the final surgical result.

- The general surgical pack for a routine surgery consists of the following instruments and surgical apparel.

General surgical Kit/pack

B. P. handle, Scissors, Rat tooth tissue forceps, Allies tissue forceps, Towel clamps, Mosquito hemostats, Artery forceps, Needle holder, Suture needles, Surgical gloves, Surgical gown, mask, cap, Drapes and Gauze sponges.

Note : special instruments needed for any operation should be sterilized along with general surgical pack or sterilized separately. The number of instruments varies according to type of surgery. Eg: orthopedic surgery.

Sterilization

General surgical pack should be sterilized in an autoclave at 15 pounds pressure for 15 mins at 121° C.

2. Preparation of the owner

Owners should be well informed about the outcome of the surgical procedure so that they can make up their mind before handling the critical situation. Consent has to be taken from the owner concerned to anesthetic risk, surgical risk and post operative complication before performing the surgical procedure.

3. Patient stabilization

Patient should be stabilized with intravenous fluids like Ringers Lactate, 5% dextrose, If required emergency drugs like steroids can be administered depending on the condition of the patient on which surgery has to be performed.

4. General preparation of patients

Fasting

- Food withheld for 12 hrs before surgery to minimize the potential for vomiting and aspiration during anesthesia but in case of intestinal surgeries minimum of 24 hrs fasting is necessary.
- Water should be restricted 3-4 hrs before surgery.

- Large Animal: 48-72 hours withdraw feed & 24 hours withdraw liquid food/water.

  This is to prevent vomition during anesthesia (because of relaxation of oropharangeal & cardia sphincter) it may enter into trachea leads to aspiration; it again leads to choke and death.
- Bladder may be expressed under anesthesia or emptied by catheterization.

Surgical site preparation

- Excessively soiled patient should be bathed before surgery to avoid contamination of the operating room and the surgical site.
- Skin and hair of the animals are a reservoir for bacteria and are recognized as a significant source of contamination and post surgical wound infections.
- Thus skin preparation techniques kill surface bacteria but do not sterilize the skin completely, because approximately 20% of the bacteria reside within deeper skin structures and are inaccessible to disinfectant solutions.
- Steps include **Hair removal** from the proposed surgical site and adjacent areas, either by shaving/clipping the hairs.
- **Cleaning and disinfection** of the area by QAC – Benzalkonium chloride, benzethonium chloride or any antiseptic solutions.

Restraint, Positioning and draping of the patient

- Positioned such that easy access to the proposed surgical site.
- Should be comfortable to the patient and the surgeon.
- Should not compromise superficial nerves and peripheral circulation.
- Should allow adequate access for monitoring
- When positioning is satisfactory the patient is secured by ropes, sand bags, troughs, adhesive tape or vacuum activated positioning bags to minimize movement during surgery.
- Aseptic draping of the surgical site: isolates the surgical site from non-sterile area and provides a sterile working area for the surgeon.

5. Preparation of surgeon and surgical team

Mental preparation

- Surgeon should review surgical procedure before surgery,
- Review the anatomy of the part to be operated.

Physical preparation

- Surgeon should have proper team consists of those people performing surgery, anesthesia, assistants and observers.
- Should have proper instruments and equipments
- Should evaluate patient and environment
- Surgeon should avoid carrying **infection to patient**, repeated scrubbing with carbolic soap, tincture iodine, 70% alcohol is required.
- Thoroughly wash hands, finger nails clipped, sweat drops to be avoided.

Preparation of the surgical team

- Surgical personnel are a major cause of **microbial contamination** during surgery;
- Careful preparation of surgical team and non-sterile personnel avoidence reduces bacterial numbers in the surgical room but doesn't eliminate them.
- To minimize contamination during surgery, strict guidelines should be followed regarding **surgical attire** of all surgical room personnel.
- All persons entering the operating room suite, regardless of whether a surgery is in progress or not, should be appropriately clothed.
- To minimize microbial contamination from the operating room personnel, **scrub clothes** should be worn in the operating suite.
- Other surgical attire includes hair coverings, masks, shoe covers, gowns and gloves. Even when surgery is not in progress; caps and masks should be worn in the surgical suite.

- The surgical team should wear the face mask and cap before scrubbing of their hands, while the animal is being prepared for surgery,
- The Surgeon and the Assistant surgeon **scrub** themselves before putting on the sterile gown and gloves.
- The hands are scrubbed in an orderly manner. First the arms and hands are washed with soap and water and then with detergent.
- The fingers and the thumb should be brushed with sterile brush systematically then the palm and back of the hand and finally the four surfaces of the arm up to the elbow.
- The hand and arm are then rinsed and the opposite hand and arm are similarly scrubbed and rinsed. Each hand and arm are scrubbed and rinsed for a minimum of 4 times.
- After scrubbing, 70% isopropyl or ethyl alcohol is poured over hands and arms. The excess of fluids should be allowed to drip from the elbows before drying with a sterile towel. First palms are dried and then the elbows.
- The sterile gown followed by gloves is put on after final scrubbing of hands and arms.

Surgical team and its conduct

Each surgical team consists to 3 or 4 members in group. Work and assignment of duties as follows :

Surgeon

- Is the **captain of the surgical team** and performs surgical operation.
- Is assisted by the assistant surgeons as and when needed.
- Uses **hand signals** as far as possible or talks slowly for necessary requests.
- should possess qualities of an ideal surgeon i.e., one who is thoughtful, kind, forgiving, understanding, quiet, controlled, foresighted and gentle.

Assistant surgeon- may be one or two persons, the primary responsibilities are:

- Assist the surgeon during operation.
- Prepares and drapes the surgical field of operation.
- Keeps operative field **free of visual obstructions**, particularly blood and clots.
- Should remember to **blot the tissues** instead of wiping them.
- Avoids accumulation of instruments, soiled sponges, remnants of sutures, abdominal packs etc, near the operative field.
- Keeps constantly in mind little details which help the surgeon and tries to help the surgeon in all possible way.

Anesthetist - primary duties are:

- Prepares and administers pre-anesthetics and the anesthetic and maintains close attention on animal during anesthesia.
- Keeps a proper anesthetic record.
- Maintains record of respiration, pulse, its quality and strength and temperature etc.
- Keeps the animal in recovery room after surgery till it recovers completely from anesthesia.

Important

- The successful completion of entire procedure requires co-ordination by all members of surgical team.
- The operation can be finished in a shorter time with a slow surgeon than with a surgeon operating with disrupted uncontrolled group.

4

Asepsis and Antisepsis

Asepsis is the absence of pathogenic microbes or infection on living tissue or environment i.e. A state of being free from pathogenic organisms.

Antisepsis

The process of destructing disease causing organism to prevent infection is called antisepsis. The drugs used to prevent growth of infectious microorganisms on living tissue are called antiseptics.

Sterilization

The process of destroying all micro-organism by chemicals, physical agents (heat, irradiation) is called steralization. Only inanimate objects can be rendered entirely sterile.

Application of Asepsis, Antisepsis in Veterinary Surgery

About 5% of small animal which undergo surgery inspite of extensive measures, they develop infection. The impact of infection ranges from minor to life threatening illness.

Therefore understanding factors which avoids wound infection is essential by following measures.

1. Strict adherence to Aseptic technique.
2. Proper sterilization of operation theatre.
3. Hygienic preparation of surgical team and its surrounding.

Disinfectants: are agents which destroy pathogenic microbes, may not inactive all viruses and spore forming bacteria. Disinfection refers to use of germicidal substances on inanimate objects. Operation tables and animal preparation room is disinfected routinely.

Antiseptics: use of antimicrobials or chemicals on living tissue. Suitable antiseptics are used to clean the surgical area after shaving and cleaning the area.

Operation theatre: It is sterilized by Irradiation (UV rays) and also disinfected using suitable disinfectants.

Surgical instruments: are sterilized by autoclaving.

Suture materials: using chemical sterilization.

Surgical gowns: by autoclaving:

Preparation of the animal: The animal part to be operated or having wound should be thoroughly washed and shaved. Then wound is washed with antiseptic and then area to be operated is draped. The surgical area can be cleaned with surgical spirit followed by povidone iodine.

Sterilization of Surgical Materials and Instruments

Sterilization is a process of complete elimination of microorganism (both vegetative forms of bacteria and spores).

Methods of Sterilization

1. Physical
2. Chemical

1. Physical method

A) Heat-moist heat (steam sterilization), Dry heat (hot air oven), Boiling Water and Flame.

B) Irradiation-UV rays, gamma rays, beta rays.

C) Filters (Bacterial and viral proof).

2. Chemical method

- Ethylene oxide gas and beta propiolactone gas.
- Formalin as gas sterilization & in solution as formaldehyde.

- Iodine and its compounds (Tincture iodine, povidone iodine)
- Quaternary ammonium compounds (zephrin chloride)
- Chlorinated compounds (Hypochlorite, Dakin'solution etc.)
- Coal tar derivatives (phenol, cresol)
- Detergents (cetrimide, chlorhexidine)
- Alchohol (70% methyl alcohol, Isopropyl alcohol)
- Oxidizing agents (H_2O_2, $Kmno_4$)

A. Heat : Heat destroys bacteria by coagulating its proteins.

Moist heat : Autoclaving (steam under pressure)- direct steam contact is the basis of steam sterilization. An autoclave is an apparatus for achieving sterilization by steam under pressure. It is fitted with automatically regulated pressure gauze and can withstand at least 60 pound pressure per square inch. A temperature of 121 ^{0}c at 15 lb pressure for 15 minutes is sufficient to destroy vegetative cells and spores. All surgical instruments in a surgical pack are sterilized by autoclaving.

Dry heat (Hot air oven) : Used for sterilization of substances which cannot be steam sterilized e.g.oils-mineral oil, linseed oil, paraffin, powder, glass wares.

Dry heat sterilization done at 160 ° C for 1 hr or 180 ° C for 20 - 30 minutes.

Infrared ovens are also used for dry sterilization.

Temperature is attained very quickly 180 °C for 10 minutes.

Boiling water : Not destructive to spores, however addition of sodium bicarbonate to 2% solution is effective for sterilization & requires 5 minutes to kill spores. Boiling water affects the sharp edges of instruments and destructive to rubber goods and glasswares.

Flame : Used for wire loops, probes, teat dilators, teat canula, smalltray, etc.

The instruments to be sterilized are to be kept in a large stainless steel tray. Methylated spirit 5-10 ml is poured over the surface and ignited. Care should be taken that fire may not spread. Stainless steel tray should be dry and if large, tilted slightly during flaming.

B. Irradiation : Sunlight has a powerful germicidal action and exposure for sufficient time will produce sterilization. The action of sun light is mainly due to contents of ultraviolet light having a wave length of 300-400 nm. The ultraviolet rays are absorbed by nucleic acid and results in death of the cell. The ultraviolet rays are produced artificially by mercury vapour lamps and used for sterilization of environment of the operating rooms and are not deep penetrating, they act on surface only. It is important to protect eye by glasses, as excessive exposure of the cornea to the ultraviolet causes severe irritation.

The shorter electromagnetic wavelength atomic rays (X-rays, gamma rays) causes ionization of the living or nonliving matter and the electron is knocked out of one molecule and gained by another. Thus both become ions of high chemical reactivity capable of causing biological damage or death. These rays are deep penetrating and used to sterilize disposable polythene, plastic catheters(heat sensitive materials).

C. Bacterial/viral filters

The bacterial and viral proof ultrafine sintered glass and membrane filters of pore size not exceeding 1nm are used for filtration of liquids which are heat sensitive. Most satisfactory filters are made of unglazed porcelain, sintered glass or nitrocellulose.

Chemical

Ethylene oxide: (Gas sterilization)

The ethylene oxide, a colorless highly inflammable water soluble gas, is used to sterilize instruments which are sensitive to heat. The time required for sterilization varies with the concentration of the gas, higher the concentration shorter the time. Rubber goods and the items which are eroded by steam like sharp eye instruments, polyethylene catheters, cytoscopes, stethoscope, stomach tubes, electric cords, nerve stimulator etc can be sterilized by gas.

Formalin

Formalin kills spores readily. The gas is derived from the Para formaldehyde tablets which are placed in a gas tight chambers designed for sterilization of endoxcoic bulbs, catheters and other delicate instruments which can not be boiled (sharp instruments).The tablets are heated with electric element or spirit lamp. Sterlization for 30 minutes is sufficient to kill microorganisms and its spores.

Beta propionolactone

Acts more rapidly than does either ethylene oxide or formaldehyde. The disadvantages of this gas are that it may damage painted and plastic surfaces. It has been used to sterilize hospital rooms and animal housing buildings, It is highly toxic and carcinogenic.

Iodine and its compounds

Iodine is effective in aqueous and alcoholic solution. Iodine kills the microorganisms by oxidation of proteins.

Quarternary ammonium compounds

They are surface active compounds and are cationic in nature. These Cause denaturation of cell proteins and inactivation of cell enzymes and disruption of cell membrane. Generally used in skin surface preparation and to preserve sterility of surgical instruments e.g zephiran chloride 1:1000 solution.

Chlorinated compounds

The compounds in solution containing 2.5% sodium hypochlorite are effective. used for irrigation of wounds. 3% solution of chloride of lime is used for sterilizing utensils.

Coal tar derivatives

These kill the microorganisms by coagulation of cell proteins or denaturation of proteins. Phenol 1% for 5 to 10 minutes, cresol 2% for 5 minutes are commonly used.

Chloroxenol

It is used as 5% solution for 30 minutes for sterilization of utensils.

Alcohol

It acts through their ionic action. Ethyl alcohol, 70% is sufficient to kill any microorganisms. The isopropyl alcohol is more effective; however, the alcohols do not have any action on spores.

Detergents

Soaps, cetrimide and chlorhexidine are used for skin preparation. 1% chlorhexidine and 2% cetrimide in alcohol in combination is good for skin preparation.

Mercurials

The heavy metals and their salts precipitate the cell protein through their ions. Bichloride of mercury 1:1000 or 1:2000 is used for disinfection of glass and rubber articles and thermometers.

Oxidizing agents

They include hydrogen peroxide, potassium permanganate 0.5 to 1% for hand scrubbing and 1:3000 for wound irrigation.

□□□

5

Surgical Risk and Judgement

Surgical risk is defined as "any undesirable result of surgery". A doctor may assess the individual patient's risk in order to better inform the owners and to allow consensual decisions for procedures to be undertaken. Risk assessment might allow consideration of a change in plan to reduce that individual's risk; for example, a more limited operation, modification of the planned anaesthetic technique or perioperative haemodynamic optimisation. In a more complex format, risk is assessed to allow suitable targeting of therapeutic options and decision-making with regard to treatment choices so that a suitable balance of risks, often between the possible side effects and dangers of surgery and the potential success of treatment, can be made. Implicit in risk assessment for the individual is the intention of subsequent action to achieve risk reduction, but as already noted this is often not achievable.

Judgement & Decision-making : Making informed and timely decisions regarding assessment, diagnosis, surgical management, follow-up, health maintenance and promotion. Principles to be followed is to recognize and articulate problems to be addressed, Initiates balanced discussion of options, pros and cons with relevant team members, Seeks second opinion when appropriate for surgeons or patients, Respects the patient's right for self determination.

Risks and complications of any type of surgery (very rare in healthy patients)

- Allergic reactions
- Nausea and vomiting (not uncommon after anaesthesia)

- Abnormal heart rhythm (arrhythmia)
- Heart attack (cardiac infarction)
- Airway obstruction
- Blood clots (deep venous thrombosis)
- Pulmonary embolism
- Fat embolism
- Stroke
- Brain damage
- Temporary or permanent paralysis
- Nerve damage (temporary or permanent)
- Malignant hyperthermia
- Sepsis (blood poisoning)
- Death

Specific Risks and Complications (selected procedures)

Rhinoplasty : Bleeding, swelling, bruising, asymmetry, obstruction of nasal airways It is not uncommon to have a revisional procedure (correction; 10-15% of rhinoplasties).

Blepharoplasty (eyelid correction) : Swelling, bruising, blurred vision, excessive tearing, dry eye, redness, asymmetry, ectropion (drooping of the lower lid caused by overcorrection or scarring), blindness (extremely rare; caused, for example, by bleeding behind the eye).

Liposuction : Contour irregularities, indentations, uneven areas, seroma (wound fluid collection), infection. Fat cells that are removed by liposuction do not come back. Nevertheless if gains significant weight, the remaining fat cells can grow again and store more fat.

Knee Arthroscopy : (1) Postoperative bleeding within the knee joint (2) Persistent swelling (3) Persistent pain (4) Stiffness (5) Knee ligament injury (6) Broken instruments inside the joint when performing surgery requiring open incision to remove (7) Tourniquet palsy which may cause some numbness & tingling in the foot (8) Compartment syndrome (9) Meniscal retear or failure to heal if repaired (10) Persistent muscle weakness.

Cardiac surgery : Patients with recent myocardial infarction or unstable angina, decompensated heart failure, high-grade arrhythmias, or hemodynamically important valvular heart disease (aortic stenosis in particular) are at very high risk for perioperative myocardial infarction, heart failure, ventricular fibrillation or primary cardiac arrest, complete heart block, and cardiac death.

Cosmetic surgery : Infection, Bleeding, Hematoma (blood collection, blood clot), Seroma (wound fluid collection), Skin/ tissue death (necrosis), Delayed healing, Swelling, Bruising, Poor scarring (wide, stretched or thickened scars), Numbness, tingling, Asymmetry, Irregularities, dimples, tuckers.

The Safe Surgery Saves Lives programme aims to improve surgical safety and reduce the number of surgical deaths and complications in four ways:

1. by giving clinicians, hospital administrators and public health officials information on the role and patterns of surgical safety in public health
2. by defining a minimum set of uniform measures or 'surgical vital statistics', for national and international surveillance of surgical care
3. by identifying a simple set of surgical safety standards that can be used in all countries and settings and are compiled in a 'surgical safety checklist' for use in operating rooms; and
4. by testing the checklist and surveillance tools.

Surgical Resources and Environment

Trained personnel, clean water, consistent light source, consistent suction, supplemental oxygen, functioning surgical equipment and sterile instruments.

Prevention of Surgical Site Infection can be done by Hand washing, Appropriate and judicious use of antibiotics, Antiseptic skin preparation, Atraumatic wound care, Instrument decontamination and Sterility.

Safe Anaesthesia can be done by Presence of a trained anaesthesia professional, Anaesthesia machine and medication, safety check of Pulse oximetry, Heart rate monitoring, Blood pressure monitoring, Temperature monitoring.

Safe Surgical Teams needs Improved communication, Correct location of surgical site and procedure Informed consent, Availability of all team members, Adequate team preparation and planning for the procedure Confirmation of animal allergies.

The aim of the working groups is to identify potential standards for improvements in four areas: *safe surgical teams*, by promoting communication among team members to ensure that each preparatory step is accomplished in a timely and adequate fashion with an emphasis on teamwork; *safe anaesthesia*, by appropriate patient monitoring and advance preparation to identifypotentially lethal anaesthetic or resuscitation problems before they cause irreversible harm; *prevention of surgical site infection*, through antisepsis and control of contamination at all levels of patient care; and *measurement of surgical services*, by creating public health metrics to measure provision and basic outcomes of surgical care.

The Safe Surgery Saves Lives Challenge is guided by three principles. The first is simplicity. An exhaustive list of standards and guidelines might create a package that would improve patient safety, but such comprehensiveness would be difficult to implement and convey and would probably face significant resistance. The appeal of simplicity in this setting cannot be overstated. Uncomplicated measures will be the easiest to institute and can have profound effects in a variety of settings. The second principle is wide applicability. Focusing on a specific resource milieu would reduce the number of issues (e.g. minimum equipment standards for resource-poor settings), but the goal of the challenge is to reach all environments and settings, from resource rich to resource poor, so that all Member States can be involved. Furthermore, regular failures occur in every setting and environment and are amenable to common solutions. The third is measurability. Measurement of impact is a key component of the Second Challenge. Meaningful metrics must be identified, even if they relate only to surrogate processes, and they must be reasonable and quantifiable by practitioners in all contexts. If the three principles of simplicity, wide applicability and measurability are followed, the goal of successful implementation will be feasible.

Surgical care is complex and involves dozens of steps which must be optimized for individual patients. In order to minimize unnecessary loss of life and serious complications, operative teams have 10 basic, essential objectives in any surgical case:

1. The team will operate on the correct patient at the correct site.
2. The team will use methods known to prevent harm from administration of anaesthetics, while protecting the patient from pain.
3. The team will recognize and effectively prepare for life-threatening loss of airway or respiratory function.
4. The team will recognize and effectively prepare for risk of high blood loss.
5. The team will avoid inducing an allergic or adverse drug reaction for which the patient is known to be at significant risk.
6. The team will consistently use methods known to minimize the risk for surgical site infection.
7. The team will prevent inadvertent retention of instruments or sponges in surgical wounds.
8. The team will secure and accurately identify all surgical specimens.
9. The team will effectively communicate and exchange critical information for the safe conduct of the operation.
10. Hospitals and public health systems will establish routine surveillance of surgical capacity, volume and results.

Five step process similar to the Universal Protocol to prevent wrong-site surgery:

Step 1 : Check that the consent form or procedure request form is correct.

Step 2 : Mark the site for the surgery or other invasive procedure.

Step 3 : Confirm identification with the patient.

Step 4 : Take a 'team time out' in the operating theatre, treatment or examination area.

Step 5 : Ensure appropriate and available diagnostic images.

Prevention and surveillance of surgical site infections: The Study on the Efficacy of Nosocomial Infection Control (SENIC) showed that about 6% of all nosocomial infections can be prevented with minimum intervention. Simple methods that can be used to limit risk include:

complete assessment of all surgical patients preoperatively, reduced preoperative hospitalization, evaluation and treatment of remote infections, weight reduction (for obese animals), administration of appropriate and timely antimicrobial prophylaxis, confirmation of proper asepsis and antisepsis of skin and instruments, maintenance of meticulous surgical technique and minimization of tissue trauma, maintenance of normothermia during surgery, shortened perating time and effective wound surveillance.

Definitions of surgical site infection: Surgical site infection is divided into two main groups, incisional and organ–space. Incisional infections are further subdivided into superficial (skin and subcutaneous tissue) and deep (deep soft tissue such as fascia and muscle layers). Organ–space surgical site infection involves any part of the anatomy other than the incision that is opened or manipulated during an operation.

The criteria for the different sites of infection are given below.

Superficial incisional surgical site infection: Infection occurs at the incision site within 30 days of surgery and involves only skin or subcutaneous tissue at the incision and at least one of the following:

1. Purulent drainage from the superficial incision.
2. An organism isolated by culturing fluid or tissue from the superficial incision;
3. Deliberate opening of the wound by the surgeon because of the presence of at least one sign or symptom of infection (pain, tenderness, localized swelling, redness or heat), unless the wound culture is negative; or
4. Diagnosis of superficial incisional surgical site infection by the surgeon or attending Physician.

The following conditions are generally not reported as surgical site infection :

1. Stitch abscess with minimal inflammation and discharge confined to the points of suture penetration;
2. Infection of an episiotomy site;
3. Infection of a neonatal circumcision site; or
4. Infected burn wound.

Deep incisional surgical site infection: Infection occurs at the site of operation within 30 days of surgery if no implant (non-human-derived foreign body permanently placed in the patient during surgery) is left in place and within 1 year of surgery if an implant is left in place. In addition, infection appears to be related to surgery and involves deep soft tissue (muscle and fascia layers) and atleast one of the following:

1. Purulent drainage from deep incision but not from the organ–space component of the surgical site;
2. Wound dehiscence or deliberate opening by the surgeon when the patient has fever (> 38 °C) or localized pain or tenderness, unless the wound culture is negative.
3. An abscess or other evidence of infection involving the deep incision seen on direct examination during surgery, by histopathological examination or by radiological examination; or
4. Diagnosis of deep incisional surgical site infection by the surgeon or attending physician.

Organ–space surgical site infection: Infection occurs within 30 days of surgery if no implant (non-human-derived foreign body permanently placed in the patient during surgery) is left in place and within 1 year of surgery if an implant is left in place. In addition, infection appears to be related to surgery and involves any part of the anatomy other than the incision that is opened or manipulated during an operation and at least one of the following:

1. Purulent drainage from a drain placed through a stab wound into the organ–space;
2. An organism isolated from an aseptically obtained culture of fluid or tissue in the organ or space;
3. An abscess or other evidence of infection involving the organ or space seen on direct examination during surgery, by histopathological examination or by radiological examination; or
4. Diagnosis of an organ–space surgical site infection by the surgeon or attending physician.

Current Recommendations of Agents for Surgical prophylaxis

Procedure Agents

Colectomy - Cefotetan, cefoxitin, cefazolin plus metronidazole, ampicillin/sulbactam or ertapenem; metronidazole combined with an aminoglycoside, a quinolone or trimethroprim/sulfamethoxazole, or clindamycin combined with an aminoglycoside, a quinolone, aztreonam or trimethroprim/sulfamethoxazolea.

Other gastrointestinal surgery - Cefotetan, cefoxitin, cefazolin or cefuroximeb.

Hysterectomy - Cefotetan, cefoxitin, cefazolin or cefuroxime, cefazolin plus metronidazolec. Vascular and cardiac surgery - Cefazolin or cefuroxime, penicillinase-resistant penicillins such asoxacillin and cloxacillin, or vancomycin or clindamycin.

Total joint replacement - Cefazolin or cefuroxime or a penicillinase-resistant penicillin.

Minimizing contamination in the operating room

1. Disinfection of surfaces: The surfaces in operating rooms should be kept clean by the use of water, detergent and wiping. keeping them clean should be enough for safety.
2. Surgical attire: The use of masks that cover the mouth and nose, hair-coverings such as caps, sterile surgical robes and impermeable sterile gloves is standard for surgical teams.
3. Sterilization is the process by which an item is purged of all microorganisms and spores. The use of sterile materials for surgery is considered standard practice internationally.

Recommendations to be done during surgery

1. A full count of sponges, needles, sharps, instruments and miscellaneous items (any other item used during the procedure and is at risk of being left within a body cavity) should be performed when the peritoneal, retroperitoneal, pelvic or thoracic cavity is entered.
2. The surgeon should perform a methodical wound exploration before closure of any anatomical cavity or the surgical site.

3. Counts should be done for any procedure in which sponges, sharps, miscellaneous items and instruments could be retained in the animal. These counts must be performed at least at the beginning and end of every eligible case.

Counts should be recorded, with the names and positions of the personnel performing the counts and a clear statement of whether the final tally was correct. The results of this tally should be clearly communicated to the surgeon.

❑❑❑

6

Management of Shock and Haemorrhage

Shock

Clinical condition characterised by decreased blood flow to vital organs due to imbalance between the size of vascular blood and effective circulatory volume and inability of the body tissue to metabolise the nutrients.

Aetiology and classification

1. **Hypovolemic shock**: tremendous reduction in circulatory volume. This can occur due to haemorrhage during surgery, trauma or severe dehydration, loss of fluid through different routes. This is the most commonly occurring shock.
2. **Cardiogenic shock**: when heart is not in a position to act as a pump.
3. **Obstructive shock**: referred to condition where a primary cause is an obstruction in flow of blood. Can occur in Gastric Dilatation and Vulvulus in dogs and acute tympany-cattle.
4. **Distributive shock**: here circulatory volume remains same and vascular space is increased. Occurs when normal tones of vessels are lost, dilation of vessels and subsequent pooling of blood in peripheral area. Generally its called as **Vasogenic shock.** This can occur in anaphylaxis and septicaemia.
5. **Septic shock**: here due to effect of organism or toxins dilation of blood vessels take place which causes pooling of blood in peripheral tissues. Similar effect in toxaemia or septicaemia, cells

of vital organs may fail to perform the normal metabolic functions despite of availability of oxygen.

Another type of classification

Primary shock: develops immediately after injury or trauma

Secondary shock: develops after 1 hour or later.

Another classification

Reversible/ compensated shock: patient can be brought back to normal levels by body mechanisms or by treatment

Irreversible/ uncompensated shock: cannot be brought back to normal level despite of treatment.

Causes of shock

a) Severe haemorrhage
b) Trauma/severe external violence/extensive injury
c) Burns-there will be effusion of fluids
d) Rough handling of viscera during surgery
e) Toxaemia associated with bacterial and other toxins
f) Bacterial infections
g) Anaphylactic reaction
h) Drugs causing cardiac suppression.

Effects of shock in various organs

Haemodynamic system

- Reduction in arterial BP
- Pulse rate: initially increased and later falls.
- RBC and WBC count increased
- pH systemic acidosis due to hypoxia
- Viscosity increases due to loss of fluid

Endocrine System : Catecholamines will be released, stimulation of glucagon and inhibition of insulin, catecholamines stimulate production of ACTH and it causes release of aldosterone from adrenal cortex and causes ADH release.

Clinical symptoms

General appearance: eyes sunken and mucous membrane will be dry and pale, cold sweating, yawning, and patient will be in a state of prostration and collapse. Vomiting and partial or complete unconsciousness. Cold extremities, superficial veins will be collapsed. Capillary refill time will be prolonged. Chyne stroke respiration is also seen in terminal periods.

Treatment

A. Replacement therapy/substitution therapy

Replacement of lost blood volume is the most important treatment especially in hypovolemic shock. Several agents are used for substitution

1. Whole blood: transfusion from a healthy animal of same species. Blood transfusion can be done in 2 ways
   a) Direct: vein of donor is catheterised and connected to vein of recipient and blood is allowed to flow through gravitational form. Disadvantage is that there won't be any control over the volume that is transfused.
   b) Indirect: blood collected from donor and stored in bags/ bottles containing anticoagulant then transfused to recipient later. Usually transfusion rate is 5.5 ml/kg.
2. Plasma: remove blood components by coagulations and centrifugation and can be administered. Any fluid that is given for replacement therapy is known as plasma volume expanders/extenders.

   They are of 2 types: colloids and crystalloids
   The life of crystalloids are very short, it will be filtered and afterwards will be removed by kidney. Commonly used agents are 0.9% normal saline or DNS, RL, ringers solution etc.

   Colloids generally have long chain carbohydrate like dextrans. Advantages are it will not be easily filtered by kidney. So high life and can be there for a longer time.

Substitution therapy continues till pulse rate is returned to normal. Minimum dose rate is 10 ml/kg and can be increased upto 90 ml/kg for a period of 24 hours depending on necessity.

B. Ventilation: maintenance of respiration with positive ventilators. Administration of oxygen will help to replace tissue damage,

C. Counteracting acidosis: administration of sodium bicarbonate or lactated ringers solution.

D. Drugs which promote cardiovascular function: like adrenaline, digitalis, dopamine etc.

E. Control of sepsis: to control the multiplication and dissemination of organisms.

HAEMORRHAGE

Haemorrhage is defined as loss of blood from vascular system as a result of diapedesis (increased porosity of blood vessel) or rhexis (rupture of blood vessel).

Causes

- Traumatic injuries,
- Failure in clotting mechanism within normal time
- Disease of blood vessels like aneurysms
- *Spirocerca* infection diseases
- Neoplasms adjacent to blood vessel or it can cause in case of infections.

Classification

Based on origin

1. Arterial Haemorrhage: blood is bright red, forced and spurts out in a pulsating manner.
2. Venous Haemorrhage: bluish red and freely flows without any pressure.
3. Capillary Haemorrhage: blood oozes out under low pressure.

Based on occurrence

1. Primary Haemorrhage: bleeding occurring immediately after wound and at the time of injury.
2. Intermediary Haemorrhage: also known as reactionary Haemorrhage. This occurs within 24 hrs. First bleeding occurs and then stops and again the bleeding recurs. Usually occurs later due to dislodging of the clots or slipping of the ligatures.
3. Secondary Haemorrhage: occurs later than 24 hrs. Occur as a result of necrosis, ulceration and suppuration of blood vessel.

Based on extent of injury

1. Petechial Haemorrhage: very small pin head sized bleeding occurring from skin/mucosa.
2. Bruising Haemorrhage: larger areas of subcuteneous or sub-mucosal Haemorrhage.
3. Frank bleeding: also known as extra-vasation.

Based on region

1. External Haemorrhage: occurs through an open wound or natural orifices. Epistaxis, haemetemesis, hematuria, melena etc.
2. Internal Haemorrhage: bleeding occurring into natural body cavity or in newly formed cavities. Haematoma, haemarthrosis, haemothorax, haemo-peritonium etc.

Prognosis of Bleeding: Small capillary bleeding-may get arrested spontaneously by natural blood clotting mechanism. But larger bleeding may require such haemostasis otherwise there will be hypovolemia with lead to shock and death.

On most of the bleeding we can await for sometime till the body mechanism work. Natural body mechanism depends on 3 mechanisms, viz., extra-vascular, vascular and intra-vascular factors.

Extra-vascular: those concerned with location of bleeding site. Elastic nature of surrounding tissue will decrease bleeding but in areas where there is little tissue surrounding blood vessel or elasticity of tissue is reduced blood may flow freely like in Cattle milk vein and dogs ear pinna.

Vascular: vaso-constriction takes place following an injury that may arrest bleeding. If blood vessel injury is severe, Tunica interna rolls inward and vessel ends retract which act as a mechanism plug to arrest bleeding and it provides a suitable surface for aggregation of platelets and clot formation

Intra-vascular: the actual clotting mechanism. Here prothrombin is converted to thrombin converted to fibrinogen converted to fibrin and then clot formation.

Mechanical measures to control the bleeding

1. **Tourniquet**: cord tied around an extremity to control bleeding. As an emergency measure, used for short period till a permanent haemostatic mechanism is adopted. Tied above the level of bleeding especially where the vessel is in close contact with the wall. Prolonged application can cause necrosis and gangrene and also cause paralysis due to pressure on the nerves.
2. **Esmarchs bandage**: used when surgeries of extremities are performed. Here a tight elastic bandage is to be applied around the distal extremity so that blood will be driven upwards and its continued above site of surgery. Then a tourniquet is applied at that level to prevent return of blood. Then bandage is removed tourniquet will be removed after surgery.
3. **Crushing**: end of bleeding vessels will be crushed with in an artery forceps. This causes rupture of tunica interna which inturn causes platelet aggregation and clot formation and its used in small bleeding vessel.
4. **Haemostat/Artery forceps:** applying for few minutes stops bleeding from small vessels.
5. **Torsion**: end of bleeding vessel will be grasped with haemostatic forceps and twisted in its long axis.
6. **Ligation/ Suturing**: tying of end of bleeding vessel with any type of suture material to prevent bleeding. Transfixation is required in case of larger vessels to avoid slippage.
7. **Pressure**: digital pressure can be applied at the site or can be done with a cotton pad or gauze and sufficient time should be allowed for body for normal mechanism to work.

8. **Tamponade**: bleeding from a cavity can be effectively controlled by plugging it with sterilised gauze pieces. These gauze is called as tamponade
9. **Application of cold**: used where other techniques could not be applied, cold water or ice packets can be used.
10. **Thermo-cautery/electrocautery**: here a red hot iron will be applied to bleeding point. Useful in small vessels.
11. **Electrosurgery/electro-coagulation**: high frequency low voltage electricity is applied to bleeding end which causes tissue coagulation at point and arrest bleeding.

Topical haemostatics

Styptics: exert astringent effect on bleeding point. Glacial acetic acid, silver nitrate, ferric sulphate, alum, tannin, tr. Benzoin, adrenalin etc.

Systemic haemostatic agents

1. Vitamin K : dose dog: 0.5-1ml, cattle:10-20 ml
2. Calcium in the form of calcium borogluconate; 25% solution. Dogs : 5-10 ml I/v,
3. Congo red: 1% dogs: 15-20 ml I/v
4. Ergometrine and posterior extracts: contains oxytocin. Mostly used in post-parturient bleeding, cause contraction of uterus. {pitocin}
5. Ethamsylate: action by causing platelet aggregation at bleeding site and stabilises capillary wall. Dogs: 250-500 mg
6. Haemocoagulase: isolated from venom of snakes of *Bothrops atrax* and *B. Jararaca.*

□□□

7

Principles of Fluid Therapy in Surgical Patients

The aim of fluid therapy is to replace losses and maintain fluid and electrolyte balance in the body, thus allowing for normal cell and organ function.

Classification of Fluids

The fluids used in intravenous fluid therapy are generally classified into the following three groups:

1. Whole blood and blood products
2. Colloids
3. Crystalloids.

Whole blood and blood products

Whole blood is used in cases of:

- Severe haemorrhage
- Severe anemia

Blood products, colloids and crystalloids are the three main fluid types used in veterinary practice. Blood transfusion requires a suitable donor and checks for compatibility. The aim is to replace 'like with like' by choosing appropriate fluids for the condition and the expected or actual water/electrolyte losses occurring in the patient. Potassium levels should ideally be monitored and any disturbances treated as necessary.

Blood collection

Blood is collected from the donor animal using a blood collection bag containing an anticoagulant: citrate phosphate dextrose (CPD) is commonly used. The blood donor must be clinically healthy and have a normal packed cell volume. Dogs should weigh a minimum of 25 kg. Blood may only be taken from an animal for a specific patient: blood cannot be taken from a donor and then stored for use on any patient in the future. Some large establishments keep donor dogs on site but this is impractical in most practice situations due to economic and space restrictions. The donor is often a pet belonging to a member of staff or a willing client and can be called upon when needed. If blood is taken from a donor animal for a specific patient but is then *not* used (e.g. if the animal dies) or if not all the donor blood is used, surplus blood can be stored. Whole blood can be stored between 1–6°C for up to three weeks.

Blood is usually collected from dogs using a standard blood collection bag. One unit (400 mL) can be collected safely from the donor. If the primary purpose of the transfusion is administration of red cells, sight hounds (e.g. Greyhounds) that have a naturally high packed cell volume are preferred as donors. The donor dog does not usually require sedation. Blood is collected from the jugular vein and local anaesthetic may be infiltrated into the skin before venepuncture. During collection, the dog is kept in a comfortable position – sitting, standing or sternal recumbency – and the vein is raised.

The collection needle, which is preattached to the blood collection bag by the manufacturer, is placed into the vein and held firmly during collection. The bag is held below the donor and agitated gently during collection to mix the blood with the anticoagulant. Collection is continued until the bag is full: weighing the bag or identifying when it is turgid with blood assesses fullness. After the needle has been removed from the vein, a firm neck bandage is kept in place for two hours to avoid the formation of a haematoma. Blood collection from cats is also from the jugular vein and is collected into a large syringe. Donor cats may require sedation although this should be avoided unless absolutely necessary. Up to 50 mL can be collected from a large healthy cat. 1 mL of anticoagulant is drawn into the syringe for every 9 mL of blood to be collected. The cat is restrained in a sitting position or upside down in the handler's lap. The blood is collected with a large (20 G) needle using good venepuncture technique.

Cross-matching can be performed in general veterinary practice. A simple compatibility test can be performed on blood:

- Place two drops of donor blood in EDTA into 1 mL of saline and add two drops of patient serum.
- Centrifuge at a low speed for 15–30 seconds.
- Flick the tube to resuspend.
- If signs of agglutination are present this suggests incompatibility.
- This test does not test for haemolysis.

Administration of blood: Blood should be carefully warmed to 37°C prior to administration – overheating will result in agglutination and protein breakdown. Blood is administered at an initial rate of 0.25 mL/kg/hour for the first 15 minutes. Constant monitoring of the recipient during this time enables observation of any potential transfusion reaction. The rate is then increased to 20 mL/kg/hour. The total volume of blood is administered over 2–4 hours.

Giving an animal blood does involve some practical problems. If clotting factors and platelets are to be supplied, the blood must be given immediately it is taken from the donor: it cannot be stored. Incompatibility reactions are most likely in the first hour following transfusion and the patient must be monitored closely. There are numerous signs that indicate a transfusion reaction and these can vary from very mild to serious life-threatening situations. If the patient is showing any abnormal clinical signs the veterinary surgeon should be informed immediately and the transfusion stopped. The usual treatment of a blood transfusion reaction is to administer crystalloid fluids, antihistamines, antibiotics and corticosteroids.

Clinical signs associated with blood transfusion reactions

1. Urticaria
2. Hypersalivation
3. Muscle tremors
4. Tachycardia
5. Vomiting/nausea
6. Restlessness
7. Jaundice
8. Dyspnoea
9. Haemoglobinuria
10. Pyrexia
11. Facial oedema
12. Tachypnoea
13. Convulsions

Colloids

Colloids are a group of fluids containing large molecules designed to remain in the intravenous space longer than crystalloid fluids. This means that colloids are able to expand and maintain the vascular volume more effectively. Their osmotic potential is so great that colloids draw fluid out of the interstitial and intracellular spaces into the plasma, hence colloids are commonly termed ***plasma expanders***.

Colloids are used in cases of shock where cardiovascular function needs to be improved rapidly:

- Haemorrhage
- Shock
- Severe dehydration.

Following haemorrhage, colloids are sometimes administered rather than blood because obtaining a blood donor is not always easy and they avoid the possibility of a blood transfusion reaction if cross-matching is not possible or practical.

Dextrans

These are artificial colloids with a high molecular weight.

Gelatins

Gelatins are straw coloured, isotonic colloid solutions. Gelatins should be stored at room temperature. They are administered through a standard fluid administration set and intravenous catheter. The patient does not require cross-matching before administration and gelatins must not be administered with whole blood.

Plasma

Plasma is also considered in this fluid category. Whole blood can be separated, e.g. by centrifugation, into plasma and packed red cells. However, facilities for this are rarely available in general veterinary practice. When possible, it does allow the patient to receive specific treatment with plasma proteins, whilst minimising the risk of a cross reaction.

Crystalloids

Crystalloids are a group of sodium-based electrolyte fluids. They enter the extracellular fluid (ECF) and from there equilibriate with other fluid compartments in the body to restore fluid balance. The most commonly used crystalloids are similar to plasma water in composition. In patients where renal function is normal, crystalloids will be excreted in the urine.

Hartmann's (lactated Ringer's) solution: Hartmann's contains electrolytes in very similar concentrations to those in the extracellular fluid (ECF). Sodium (Na+), potassium (K+), calcium (Ca++), chloride (Cl--) and lactate are present. Hartmann's is indicated in many cases of fluid and electrolyte losses. The lactate present is metabolised to bicarbonate, and this is used in the body to overcome situations of metabolic acidosis, which occur in many clinical conditions.

0.9% sodium chloride (saline): This solution contains sodium (Na+) and chloride (Cl), but no potassium (K^+). 0.9% sodium chloride is indicated in fluid and electrolyte losses, particularly when plasma potassium levels are increased due to underlying disease and additional administration of potassium must be avoided during fluid therapy.

5% dextrose: 5% dextrose, also referred to as 5% glucose, is basically water with a small amount (50 mg/mL) of glucose added in order to make it isotonic, thus enabling it to be administered intravenously. This solution contains no electrolytes so provides the body with water and a very small amount of glucose. 5% dextrose is indicated in situations of primary water loss, where the animal is unable to take in oral fluids, and in cases of hypoglycaemia. The amount of glucose present is too little to make a significant contribution to the energy intake of the animal.

0.18% sodium chloride and 4% glucose (glucose-saline): Glucose-saline is mainly water but also has a small amount of sodium and chloride to replace daily urinary losses in the normal animal. It is used in cases of primary water loss and occasionally as a maintenance fluid, although in the latter case potassium should be added to the drip bag.

Ringer's solution: Ringer's solution contains mainly sodium, chloride and some potassium. It is indicated in water and electrolyte loss when there is also some potassium deficit. It is mainly used in cases of pyometra when severe vomiting is present. Vomiting leads to substantial losses of hydrogen and chloride which in turn produces an excess of sodium. The kidneys try to compensate for the sodium excess, which can give rise to hypokalaemia.

Darrow's solution: This solution contains sodium, chloride, and potassium in higher concentrations than Ringer's or Hartmann's. Darrow's solution is mainly indicated in cases of metabolic acidosis with potassium deficiency, e.g. persistent diarrhoea.

Hypertonic saline (7.8% or 9% sodium chloride): Hypertonic saline is under-used in small animal intravenous fluid therapy, but is more widely accepted in large animal fluid therapy. When this type of sodium chloride is administered intravenously, its high osmotic potential causes fluid from the intracellular space to move into the vascular space. This causes a sudden rapid increase in circulating volume that is needed in cases of severe hypovolaemia. Hypertonic saline is therefore indicated in situations such as: gastric dilation and volvulus (GDV), equine colic, severe haemorrhage. Typically, a 7.8% solution of hypertonic saline is administered intravenously at a rate of 4–5 mL/kg.

❑❑❑

8

Abscess, Tumors, Cyst, Haematoma, Necrosis, Gangrene and Burn

ABSCESS

It is an abnormal cavity in the tissues containing pus lined by pyogenic membrane. (fig.15)

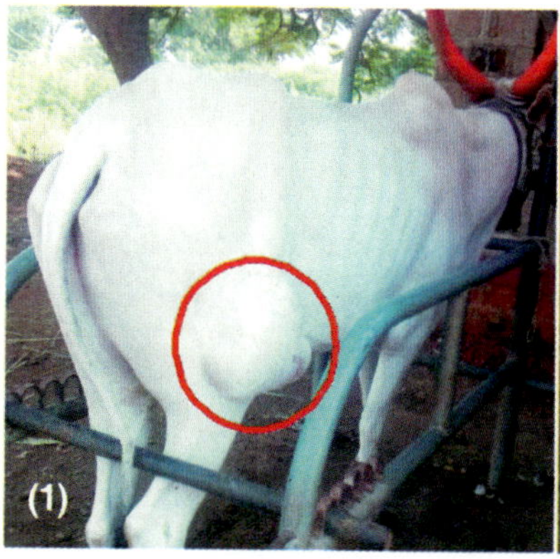

Abscess at thigh region in cattle

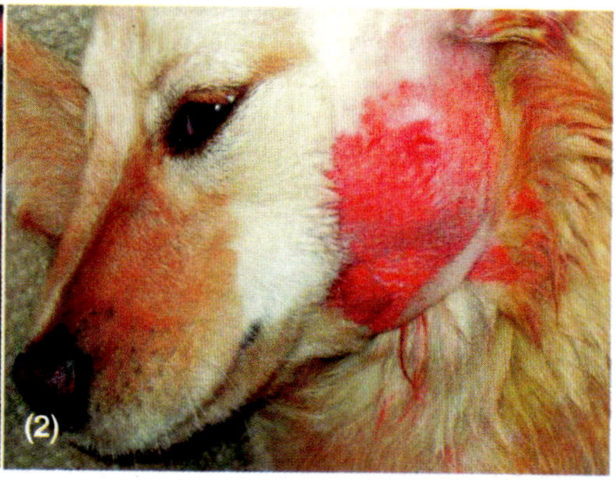

Abscess in dog

Fig.15. 1&2

Pus is the liquefied portion of the necrotic tissue with leucocytes (cellular infiltration). It is creamy in colour may be watery or cheesy. Pyogenic membrane will be present which reacts with invading organism. It is protective in nature due to humoral antibodies which prevent further spreading of abscess to the adjacent area. It is called localized abscess.

Etiology: organism like streptococci, staphylococci coli, coryne bacteria, pseudomonous etc.

Classification

1. **Acute/hot /superficial abscess:** It develops superficially, appears first as localized painful inflammatory swelling. The centre of the swelling is hard and red in color. When the abscess matures it is soft and fluctuating at the centre of the skin because skin becomes thin when the abscess is said to be "pointing" or "maturing" or ripening". In this area one could see the creamy pus, however at the periphery it is firm.
2. **Chronic/cold/deep abscess:** It develops slowly, and develops under thick layer of tissue (like fascia, muscle) give rise to pyrexia and pain on manipulation of the part. After such an abscess ruptures the pus migrates along the line of least resistence. Abscess situated closed to rectum, pharynx, larynx and spinal cord create serious functional disturbances.

Differential diagnosis

1. Cysts: develops slowly and fluctuates uniformly, no inflammatory symptoms.
2. Haematoma: usually occurs immediately after injury, crepitates on pressure.
3. Hernia: Protrusion of an organ or tissue through an opening under the skin. Contents get reduced and hernial ring can be felt.
4. Tumour: Develop slowly without inflammatory symptoms. It is hard on palpation and periphery is circumscribed.
5. Hygroma: The inflammation of the joint. Swelling in joint is seen. On exploration we get synovial fluid.
6. Oedema: It is soft doughy cold swelling and it pits on pressure.

Prognosis: Single abscess is favourable

Multiple abscesses are unfavourable.

An abscess along an air passage of pharynx, very close to nerve or blood vessel, viscinity are more dangerous.

Treatment

1. Fomentation or application of blisters (Bin iodide of mercury ointment) is advised to bring about early maturation of abscess.

2. Surgical treatment. (Lancing an abscess): "Symes abscess knife" is used for lancing an abscess.

Procedure: A sterilized symes abscess knife is boldly inserted into the pointing of abscess with the sharp cutting edge upwards. It should be as far possible in a "dependent portion" to facilitate drainage. If abscess is not pointing in dependent portion it is sometimes necessary to make another opening in dependent portion to provide drainage called counter opening. To make counter opening, a seton needle may be passed through and taken out through the dependent portion.

After opening the abscess, the content usually starts draining. The abscess cavity should be irrigated with hypertonic saline. Afterwards it is stuffed with gauze dipped in antiseptics. The gauze packs are removed after twenty four hours and then abscess cavity is irrigated with a mild antiseptic lotion.(Acriflavin 1 in 500 solution) The abscess cavity from second day onwards is packed with sterile gauze dipped in antiseptic solutions which favours drainage and absorption of fluid exudates.

Topical application of antiseptics or antibiotics in the form of ointments or dusting powder is indicated. If virulent infection is suspected, systemic use of antibiotics may also be necessary.

The normal time required for healing of an opened out abscess is usually three weeks.

TUMOR (Neoplasm): The word neoplasm means new growth. A tumour is caused by purposeless multiplication of living cells. (fig.16)

Carnivores are more susceptible than herbivores and old animals are affected more commonly than young animals.

Classification: Clinically tumours classified as :

1. Benign tumours.
2. Malignant tumours.
3. Based on histological structures tumours may be classified as fibroma, osteoma, etc.
4. Based on embryonic layer from which tumour tissue is derived, tumours are classified as epiblast, mesoblast or hypoblast.

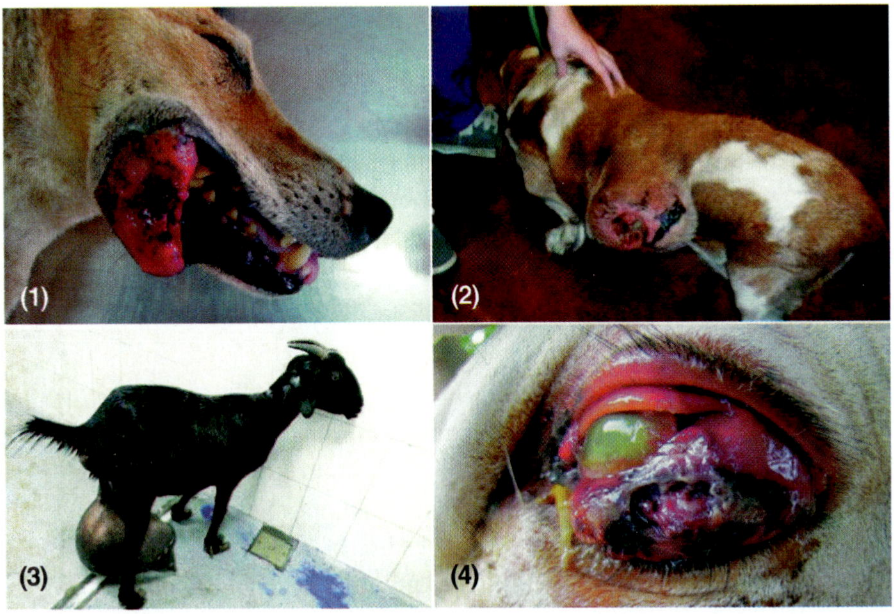

Fig.16. (1) Oral Tumour in dog (2) Ulcerated Tumour in Dog (3) Mammary gland tumour in goat (4) Squamous Cell Carcinoma in Cattle

Characteristics of tumour

1. Atypical proliferation.
2. Infiltration into surrounding tissue.
3. Destruction of invading tissue.
4. Permiation through lymphatics and blood (metastasis).

Benign Tumour	Malignant Tumour
1. Slow growing	Fast growing
2. Localized	Secondary tumour, by metastasis.
3. Adhere to skin	Do not adhere to skin
4. Do not Ulcerate	Ulcerate
5. Do not relapse after surgery.	Relapse after surgery
6. Resemble tissue origin	Do not resemble tissue origin.

Diagnosis

1. Clinical symptoms
2. Radiographs

3. Ultrasound scanner.
4. Biopsy and histopathology.
5. Exfoliative cytology.

Treatment

1. **Radical surgery**: Surgical excision of the tumour mass without leaving any tissue.
2. **Chemotherapy**.: It is taken before surgery and also after surgery.
3. **Radiation therapy**: Here low doses of radiation are applied to directly on the fast multiplying cells.
4. **Cryosurgery**: Here compressed carbon dioxide or liquid nitrogen is used to create ischemic necrosis so that mass slough off.

CYSTS

It is a non inflammatory swelling /sac with a secretory wall and its contents. Contents could be either liquid, semisolid, solid. Some time cyst contains solid structure like tooth and hair. (fig.17)

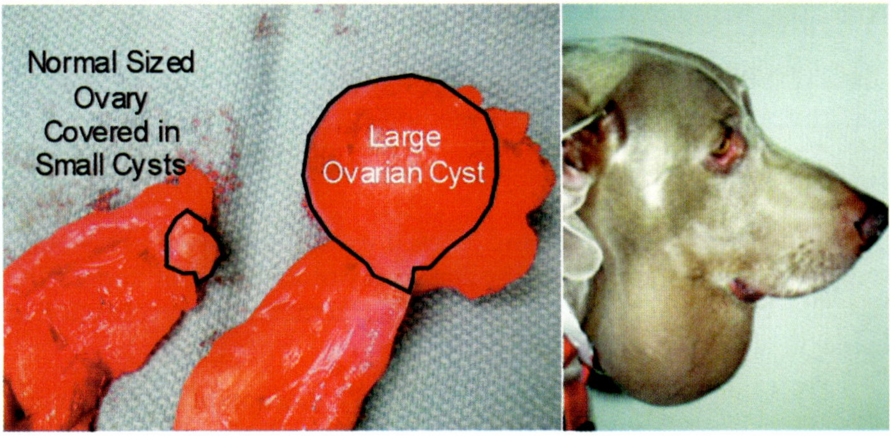

Fig.17. Cysts (1) Ovarian Cyst (2) Salivary Cyst

Classification

1. Retention cyst: arising from occlusion of duct or gland e.g. salivary cyst, ranula
2. Exudation cyst:due to accumulation of fluid in a pre existing cavity e.g. hydrocoele

3. Congenital cyst: seen at the time of birth, due to failure of an embryonic cavity to close.e.g. urachal cyst.
4. Cyst developing from misplaced embryonic tissue e.g. dermoid cyst, dentigerous cyst.
5. Encapsulation cyst formed around foreign bodies and parasites.
6. Degeneration cyst resulting from degeneration of new growth.

Diagnosis: cysts are non-inflammatory and slow in development, have well defined periphery, fluctuate uniformly if contain fluid, if contents are semisolid and hard it fluctuate enmasse. Exploratory puncture may help to confirm the diagnosis.

Treatment

1. The cyst is punctured with a trocar and canula or inoculation needle and contents are evacuated. An irritant solution like tincture iodine is then injected in to the cavity to destroy the lining membrane. During the healing process, the cavity of cyst may get obliterated.
2. The cyst may be incised to evacuate the contents. This is useful when the contents are semisolid or solid.
3. Passing a seton through the cyst.
4. Excision of cyst is the best method (Like tumour).

HAEMATOMA

It is a kind of closed wound. Closed wound is defined as a wound in which there is no break in the continuity of the skin but underlying tissues are damaged to varying degrees. Haematoma is a collection of blood in abnormal cavities. (fig.18)

A hematoma is defined as a localized collection of blood outside the blood vessels. A seroma is similar except that the fluid accumulation contains only serum without red blood cells being present.

Hematomas and seromas can occur anywhere in the body. Subdermal hematomas/seromas form under the skin and are probably the most common type of hematoma or seroma. However, hematomas and seromas can also occur within the head or brain, within other organs of the body and even on the ear (i.e., aural hematoma).

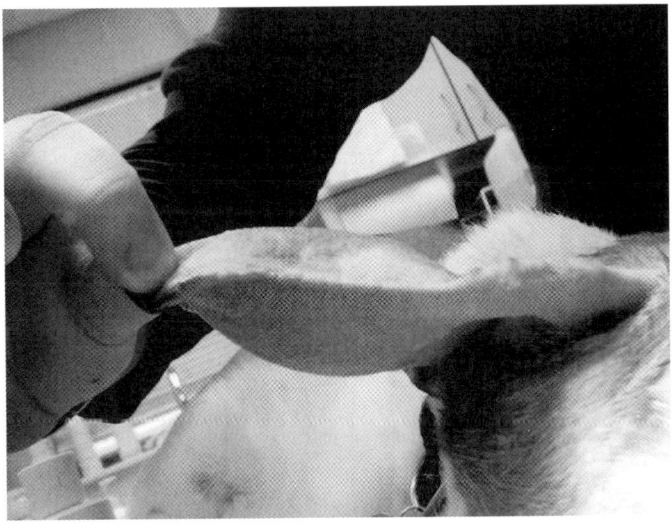

Fig.18. Aural Hematoma in dog

Symptoms will depend on the location of the hematoma or seroma

- Subdermal hematomas and seromas will result in a fluctuant swelling under the skin.
- Hematomas or seromas in the head/brain can cause a variety of symptoms, including coma, seizures and other neurological abnormalities.
- Hematomas and seromas in other organs may be asymptomatic or may cause failure or dysfunction of the organ involved.

Causes

Trauma is the most common cause of hematomas and seromas. Other causes include blood clotting abnormalities which lead to excessive bleeding.

Diagnosis

Diagnosis of a hematoma or seroma depends on the location as well. Subdermal hematomas and seromas can generally be diagnosed by physical examination coupled with evaluation of fluid withdrawn from the lesion. Hematomas and seromas in internal organs or in the brain/head may require special imaging (X-ray, ultrasound, MRI or CT scan) for diagnosis.

Treatment: Draining the cavity. We can approach the cavity with a single linear incision or S-shaped incision. The incision should be as long as that of the haematoma. Drain the contents, then scrape the inner part and apply tincture iodine. Make the skin edges smooth by clipping the edge and then apply sutures with non-absorbable material.

NECROSIS

Necrosis is a form of cell injury which results in the premature death of cells in living tissue by autolysis.

Greek word which means "death or killing"

Necrosis is caused by factors external to the cell or tissue, such as infection, toxins, or trauma which result in the unregulated digestion of cell components. In contrast, apoptosis is a naturally occurring programmed and targeted cause of cellular death.

Cellular death due to necrosis does not follow the apoptotic signal transduction pathway, but rather various receptors are activated, and result in the loss of cell membrane integrity and an uncontrolled release of products of cell death into the extracellular space.

There are six distinctive morphological patterns of necrosis

1. **Coagulative necrosis** is characterized by the formation of a gelatinous (gel-like) substance in dead tissues in which the architecture of the tissue is maintained and can be observed by light microscopy. Coagulation occurs as a result of protein denaturation, causing albumin to transform into a firm and opaque state. This pattern of necrosis is typically seen in hypoxic (low-oxygen) environments, such as infarction. Coagulative necrosis occurs primarily in tissues such as the kidney, heart and adrenal glands. Severe ischemia most commonly causes necrosis of this form.

2. **Liquefactive necrosis** (or colliquative necrosis), in contrast to coagulative necrosis, is characterized by the digestion of dead cells to form a viscous liquid mass. This is typical of bacterial, or sometimes fungal, infections because of their ability to stimulate an inflammatory response. The necrotic liquid mass is frequently creamy yellow due to the presence of dead leukocytes and is commonly known as pus. Hypoxic infarcts in the brain presents

as this type of necrosis, because the brain contains little connective tissue but high amounts of digestive enzymes and lipids, and cells therefore can be readily digested by their own enzymes.

3. **Gangrenous necrosis** can be considered a type of coagulative necrosis that resembles mummified tissue. It is characteristic of ischemia of lower limb and the gastrointestinal tracts. If superimposed infection of dead tissues occurs, then liquefactive necrosis ensues (wet gangrene)
4. **Caseous necrosis** can be considered a combination of coagulative and liquefactive necrosis, typically caused by mycobacteria (e.g. tuberculosis), fungi and some foreign substances. The necrotic tissue appears as white and friable, like clumped cheese. Dead cells disintegrate but are not completely digested, leaving granular particles. Microscopic examination shows amorphous granular debris enclosed within a distinctive inflammatory border. Granuloma has this characteristic.
5. **Fat necrosis** is specialized necrosis of fat tissue, resulting from the action of activated lipases on fatty tissues such as the pancreas. In the pancreas it leads to acute pancreatitis, a condition where the pancreatic enzymes leak out into the peritoneal cavity, and liquefy the membrane by splitting the triglyceride esters into fatty acids through fat saponification. Calcium, magnesium or sodium may bind to these lesions to produce a chalky-white substance. The calcium deposits are microscopically distinctive and may be large enough to be visible on radiographic examinations. To the naked eye, calcium deposits appear as gritty white flecks.
6. **Fibrinoid necrosis** is a special form of necrosis usually caused by immune-mediated vascular damage. It is marked by complexes of antigen and antibodies, sometimes referred to as "immune complexes" deposited within arterial walls together with fibrin.

The nucleus changes in necrosis, and characteristics of this change are determined by manner in which its DNA breaks down:

- **Karyolysis**: the chromatin of the nucleus fades due to the loss of the DNA by degradation.
- **Pyknosis**: the nucleus shrinks and the chromatin condenses.
- **Karyorrhexis**: the shrunken nucleus fragments to complete dispersal.

Treatment

- Debridement, referring to the removal of dead tissue by surgical or non-surgical means, is the standard therapy for necrosis. Depending on the severity of the necrosis, this may range from removal of small patches of skin, to complete amputation of affected limbs or organs. Chemical removal of necrotic tissue is another option in which enzymatic debriding agents, categorised as proteolytic, fibrinolytic or collagenases, are used to target the various components of dead tissue. In select cases, special maggot therapy using *Lucilia sericata* larvae has been employed to remove necrotic tissue and infection.
- Wounds caused by physical agents, including physical trauma and chemical burns, can be treated with antibiotics and anti-inflammatory drugs to prevent bacterial infection and inflammation. Keeping the wound clean from infection also prevents necrosis.
- Chemical and toxic agents (e.g. pharmaceutical drugs, acids, bases) react with the skin leading to skin loss and eventually necrosis. Treatment involves identification and discontinuation of the harmful agent, followed by treatment of the wound, including prevention of infection and possibly the use of immunosuppressive therapies such as anti-inflammatory drugs or immunosuppressants. In the example of a snake bite, the use of anti-venom halts the spread of toxins while receiving antibiotics to impede infection.

GANGRENE

Gangrene (or **gangrenous necrosis**) is a type of necrosis caused by a critically insufficient blood supply. It is potentially life-threatening condition may occur after an injury or infection, or when suffering from any chronic health problem affecting blood circulation. The primary cause of gangrene is reduced blood supply to the affected tissues, which results in cell death.

Gangrene derives from the Latin word *gangraena* and from the Greek *gangraina* which means "putrefaction of tissues".

There are different types of gangrene with different symptoms, such as dry gangrene, wet gangrene, gas gangrene, internal gangrene and necrotizing fasciitis. Treatment depends on the underlying cause, and can include resection, debridement (or, in severe cases, amputation) of the affected body parts, antibiotics, revascularization (via a vascular bypass or angioplasty), or hyperbaric oxygen therapy.

Types

Dry gangrene: is a form of coagulative necrosis that develops in ischemic tissue, where the blood supply is inadequate to keep tissue viable. Dry gangrene is often due to peripheral artery disease, but can be due to acute limb ischemia. The limited oxygen in the ischemic limb limits putrefaction and bacteria fail to survive. The affected part is dry, shrunken and dark reddish-black. The line of separation usually brings about complete separation, with eventual falling off the gangrenous tissue if it is not removed surgically, a process called autoamputation.

Dry gangrene is the end result of chronic ischemia without infection. If ischemia is detected early, when there are ischemic wounds rather than gangrene, the process can be treated by revascularization (via vascular bypass or angioplasty). However, once gangrene has developed, the affected tissues are not salvageable. Dry gangrene is seen in case of tail gangrene in cattle. (fig.19)

Wet gangrene or infected gangrene: is characterized by thriving bacteria and has a poor prognosis (compared to dry gangrene) due to sepsis resulting from the free communication between infected fluid and circulatory fluid. In wet gangrene, the tissue is infected by saprogenic microorganisms (*Clostridium perfringens* or *Bacillus fusiformis*, for example), which cause tissue to swell and emit a fetid smell. Wet gangrene usually develops rapidly due to blockage of venous (mainly) and/or arterial blood flow. The affected part is saturated with stagnant blood, which promotes the rapid growth of bacteria. The toxic products formed by bacteria are absorbed, causing systemic manifestation of sepsis and finally death. The affected part is edematous, soft, putrid, rotten and dark. Because of the high mortality associated with infected gangrene, an emergency salvage amputation has to be undertaken to limit systemic effects of the infection. It is seen in Black Quarter disease caused by clostridium organisms. (fig.19)

Gas gangrene: Gas gangrene is a bacterial infection that produces gas within tissues. It can be caused by *Clostridium*, most commonly alpha toxin producing *Clostridium perfringens*, or various non-clostridial species. Infection spreads rapidly as the gases produced by bacteria expand and infiltrate healthy tissue in the vicinity. Because of its ability to quickly spread to surrounding tissues, gas gangrene should be treated as a medical emergency.

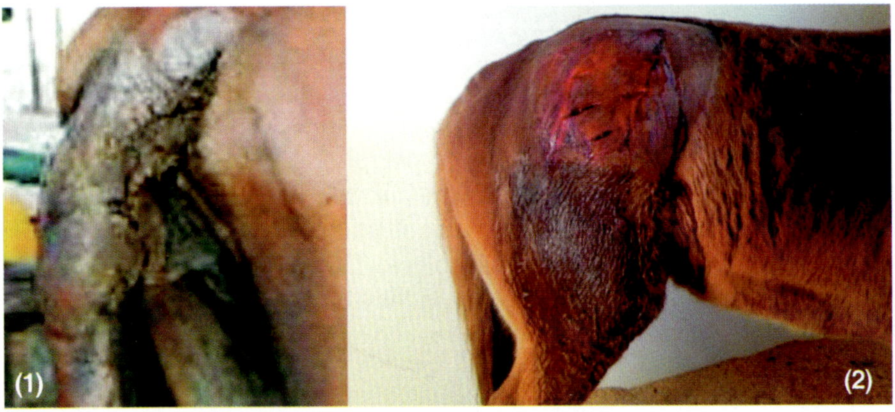

Fig.19. Gangrene (1) Dry Gangrene at tail region in cattle (2) Wet gangrene at thigh region in horse

Gas gangrene is caused by bacterial exotoxin-producing clostridial species, which are mostly found in soil, and other anaerobes such as *Bacteroides* and anaerobic streptococci. These environmental bacteria may enter the muscle through a wound and subsequently proliferate in necrotic tissue and secrete powerful toxins. These toxins destroy nearby tissue, generating gas at the same time. A gas composition of 5.9% hydrogen, 3.4% carbon dioxide, 74.5% nitrogen, and 16.1% oxygen has been reported. Gas gangrene can cause necrosis, gas production, and sepsis. Progression to toxemia and shock is often very rapid.

Complication: Sloughing, toxaemia, haemorrhage. In gangrenous mastitis in goats, the intra-cellular part gets sloughed off.

Treatment

The method of treatment is generally determined by the location of affected tissue and extent of tissue loss. The best treatment for gangrene is revascularization (i.e., restoration of blood flow) of the afflicted organ, which can reverse some of the effects of necrosis and allow healing. Other treatments include antibiotic therapy, wound care, debridement and surgical amputation.

Most amputations are performed for ischemic disease of the lower extremity. Antibiotics alone are not effective because they may not penetrate infected tissues sufficiently. Hyperbaric oxygen therapy (HBOT) treatment is used to treat gas gangrene. HBOT increases pressure and oxygen content to allow blood to carry more oxygen to inhibit anaerobic organism growth and reproduction. Growth factors, hormones and skin grafts have also been used to accelerate healing for gangrene and other chronic wounds.

BURNS

Injuries caused by heat, cold corrosive. Heat and corrosive agents causes denaturation and coagulation of proteins and cold causes burns by freezing, reduction of blood supply causes delay in healing process. Burns are the injuries caused by flame or hot solid objects. If injury is caused by a hot liquid or steam then its called as scald and this is more dangerous because it can penetrate more. Degree of injury is proportional to temperature of object and duration of contact. (fig. 20 & 21)

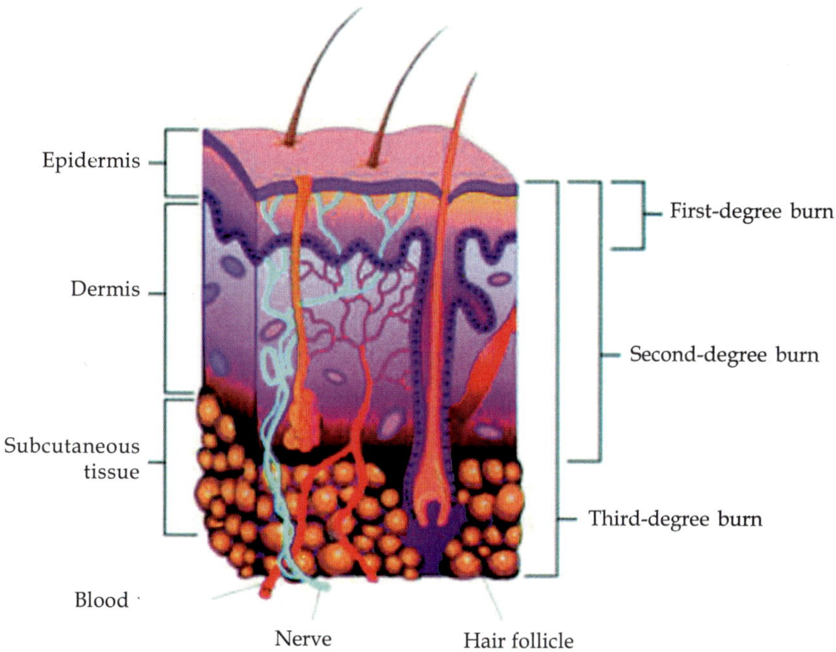

Fig. 20. Skin region showing various parts and degree of burn

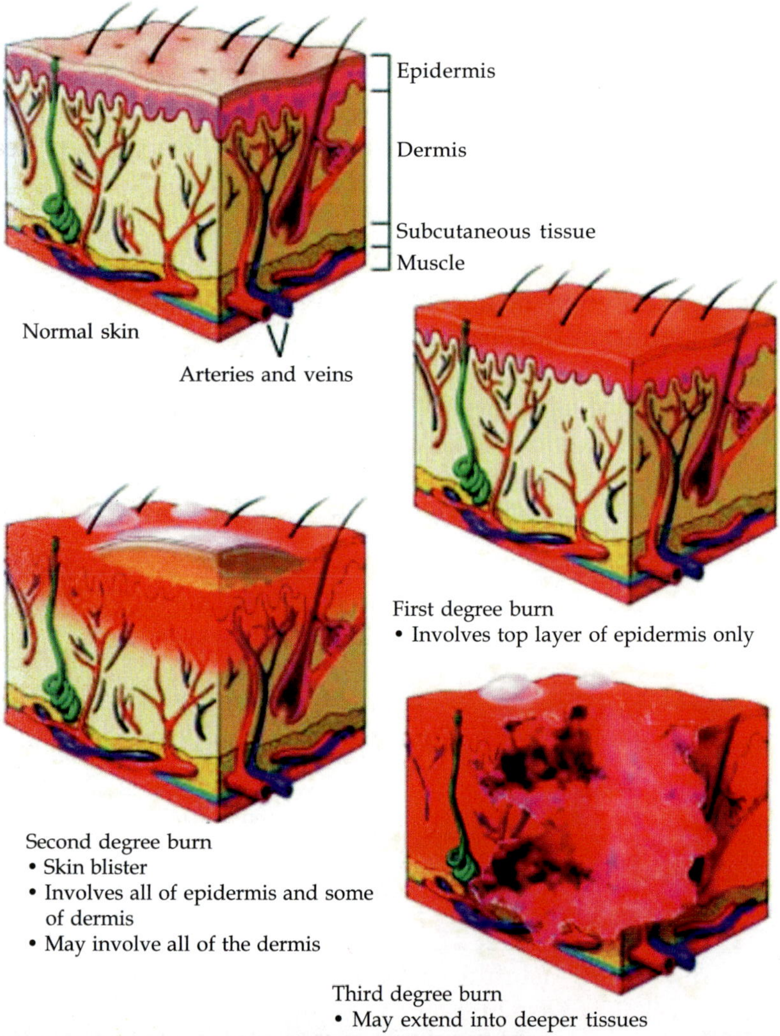

Fig.21. Skin region showing normal skin, first, second, third degree burn

Classification

1st degree: only superficial layer i.e., epidermis

2nd degree: epidermis totally lost and subcutis will not be affected

3rd degree: involves tissues like subcutis, fat and muscle and skin are totally affected.

Depth and extend of burn determine the severity.

Symptoms

1st degree: diffused swelling and sometimes vesicle formation and vesicle subside afterward.

2nd degree: formation of blisters and larger vesicles and exudation of plasma and exudation may continue for 36-42 hrs and blisters will be highly painful.

3rd degree: skin, subcutenous fat and deeper tissues are involved. Skin will be charred, hard and leathery and dark in colour and will be having bad odour. On later occasions, charred area may be sloughed off. When sloughing off of tissue takes place it is replaced by scar tissue which may appear thin, shiny and hairless. Systemically there will be pain and extensive fluid loss leading to thirst. If fluid loss is severe, animal may succumb to shock. There will be varying degree of toxaemia in absorption of toxins from damaged tissue and septicaemia may develop subsequent to secondary bacterial infection.

Treatment

Thermal burns: Depends on extent of the burn, Immediate cooling of the area is crucial. Use only cold water for 30 to 40 minutes. Do not use ice or ice packs. This may result in low body temperature or even frostbite.

1. **Superficial burns:** Hair is carefully shaved from the burn. The wound is gently cleaned with povidone iodine or chlorhexidine. Topical creams such as silver sulfadiazine are quite effective in burns. Aloe vera compounds -preserve a potent dermal vasculature to ensure tissue oxygenation & prevent progress of burn. Most of these burns heal within 3 to 5 days.
2. **Deep partial thickness burns**: Intravenous fluids are started to provide hydration and needed electrolytes - Ringer's lactate. Wounds cleaned daily with povidone iodine or chlorhexidine. Topical cream such as silver sulfadiazine is used to treat and prevent superficial infection. If over 15 percent of the body is burned, 'skin grafts is required. These burns typically heal within a few weeks.
3. **Full thickness burns**: Require extensive hospitalization and nursing care. Intravenous fluids are important in full thickness burns. Ringer's Lactate-4ml/kg/hr. Shock can occur within 1 to

2 hours of the burn. To counteract the loss of fluids, plasma transfusions are necessary or Dextrans -10-20 ml / kg /day. Antibiotics are used topically to the burn and may be used systemically. Initially, antibiotics are avoided to prevent the development of resistance bacterial strains. Anemia can occur from blood loss or early red blood cell destruction. In severe cases, blood transfusions may be needed.

Burns are painful and many burned pets are given morphine-0.25-1mg/kg tid, buprenorphine-0.01-0.02mg/kg s/c bid. Anti-inflammatory drugs-ketoprofen-2mg/kg. Steroids are not recommended.

Chemical burns: Ingesting or licking a caustic or corrosive chemical such as bleach or disinfectants. Caused by acid, alkali, gasoline or other corrosive chemicals, when they come in contact with the skin. The degree of tissue destruction depends on strength of chemical & duration of contact. Acid on the skin is neutralized by rinsing with baking soda (four tablespoons to a pint of water). Alkali is neutralized by rinsing with a weak vinegar solution (two tablespoons to a pint of water). Blot dry and apply antibiotic ointment (Furacin, Neosporin). Topical cleaning agent Glyoxide® is used . Medications such as sucralfate are used when the esophagus and stomach are involved. Sucralfate -0.5-1gm/po tid or qid.

Electrical: If burns are present in the mouth, the affected area will be cleaned and apply antibiotics. If there is fluid accumulation within the lungs, treatment with diuretics Frusemide = 2-5 mg/kg BID I/V or I/M. In shock-Intravenous fluid, oxygen should be supported.

❑❑❑

9

Wound

A wound is a break in continuity of soft tissues caused by trauma of Soft tissues-skin, muscles, subcutaneous tissues, tendons ligaments.

Classification

A. Open wound. (fig.22)

B. Closed wound.

Open wound

Break in continuity of skin.

Types

Incised wound: Caused by sharp cutting edges like knives/blades. wound edges are regular and even. damage to wound edges will be minimum. (fig.23)

Lacerated wound: Caused by tearing of tissue (barbed wire). Wound edges are torn and uneven, damage to wound edges will be more. There will be separation of wound edges from underlying tissues causing lot of pockets, may favour collection of exudates, healing will be delayed because of necrosis and sloughing off of wound edges. (fig.24)

Punctured wound: Caused by a sharp object like a nail. Opening of wound will be very small, but wound will be deep and a lot of disease infecting material will be entering into depths of wound. Such wounds are very difficult to clean. (fig.25)

Penetrating wound: These are deep wound communicating with cavities like abdomen, thorax, larynx, trachea, joints etc. caused by very sharp penetrating objects. Possibilities of vital organs getting injured. (fig.26)

Perforating wound: Wounds which passes through thickness of the tissues through two openings(one entry and one exit) e.g. Rifle wound (fig.27)

Gun shot wounds: Caused by fire arms. Here entrance will be very small and damage to underlying tissues will be extensive. (fig.28)

Abrasion wound: These are superficial wounds, characterized by mechanical removal of superficial layers of skin. These wounds are caused by scraping or friction, small capillaries will be damaged and there will be dried up clots on surface of wound.

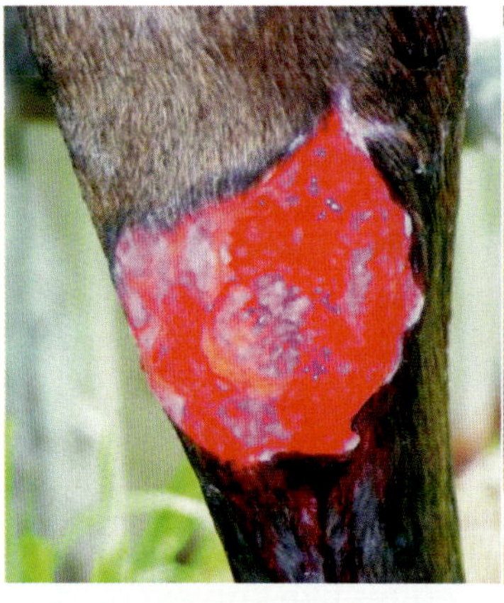

Fig.22. Open Wound

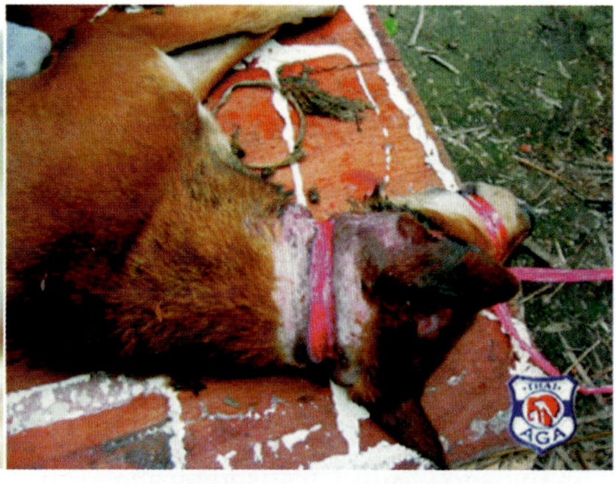

Fig.23. Incised Wound

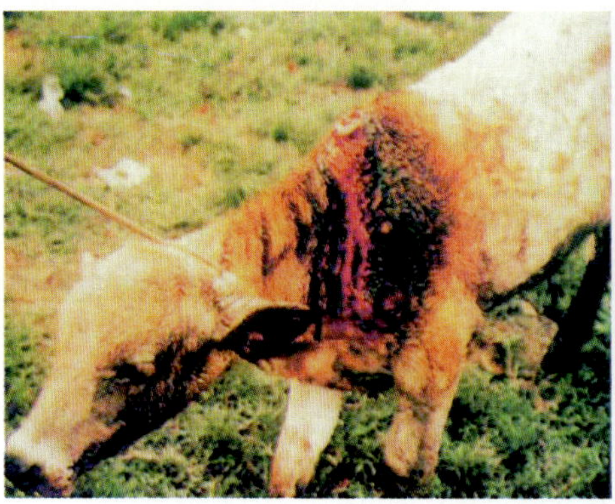

Fig.24. Lacerated Wound

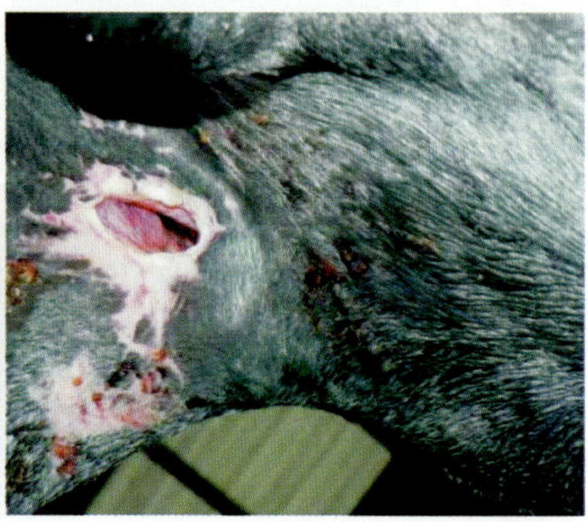

Fig.25. Punctured Wound

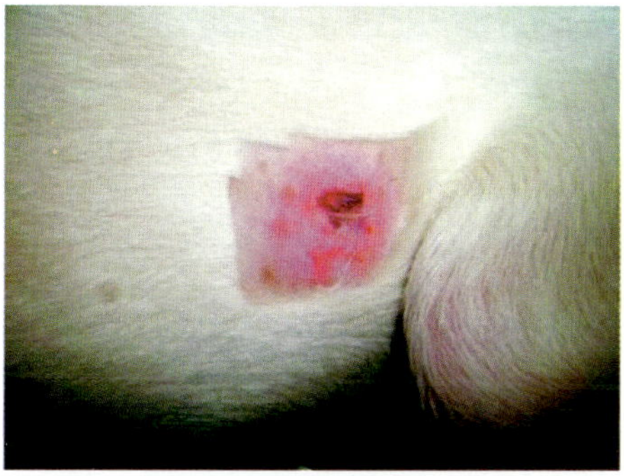

Fig.26. Penetrating Wound

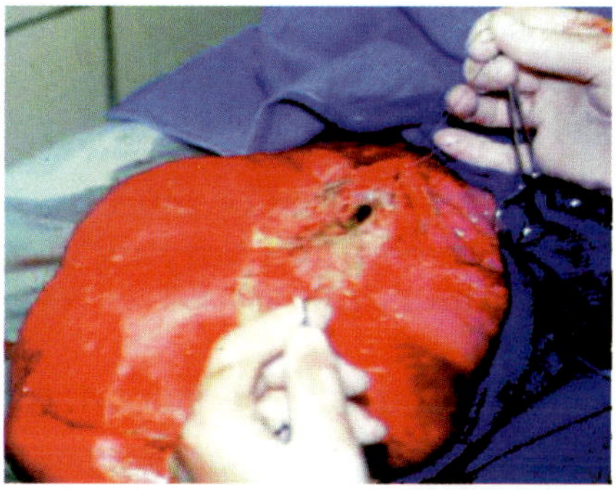

Fig.27. Perforating Wound

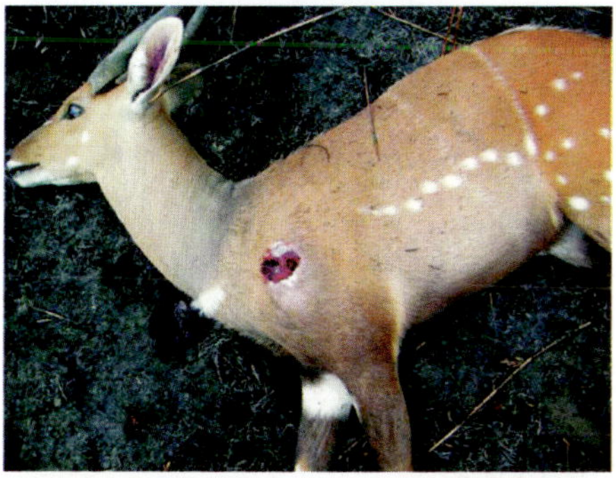

Fig.28. Gunshot Wound

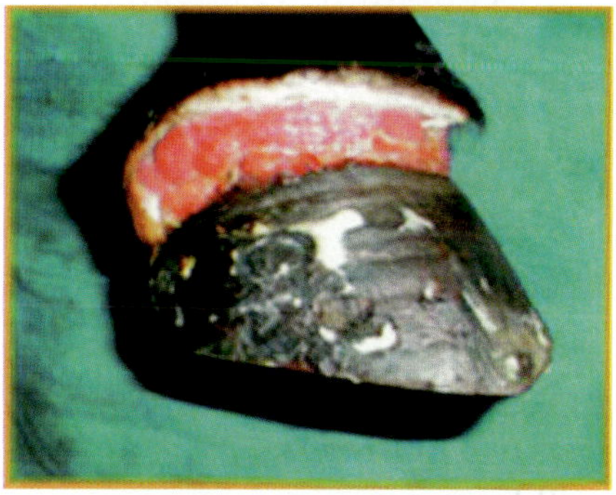

Fig.29. Avulsion Wound

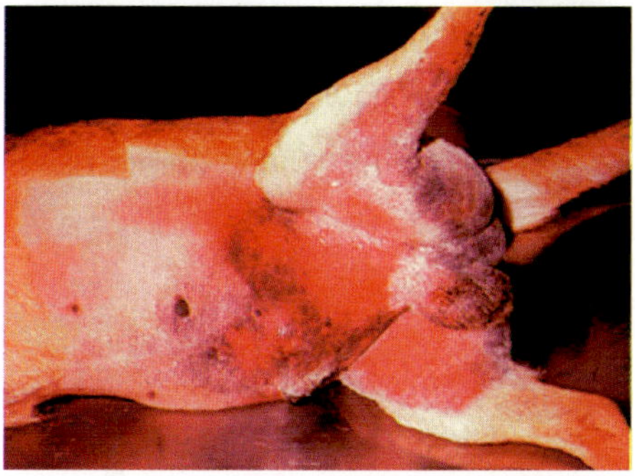

Fig. 30. Contusion Wound

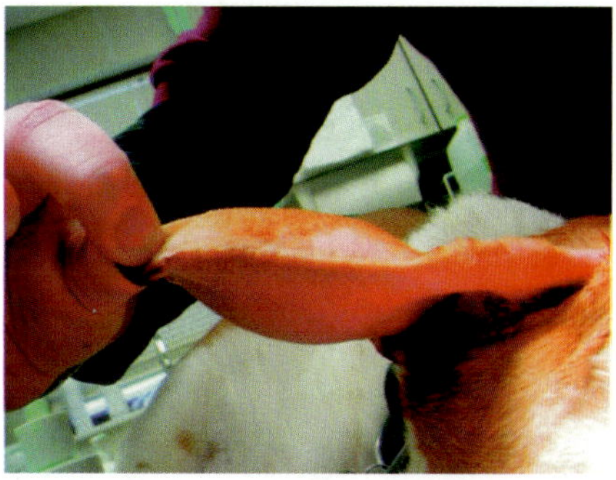

Fig.31. Hematoma Wound

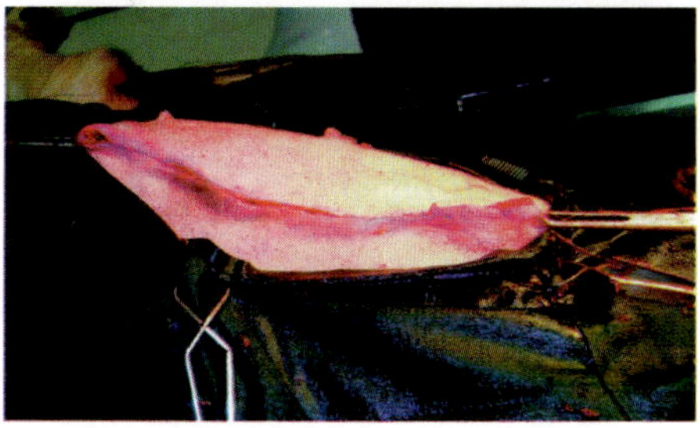

Fig.32. Aseptic Wound

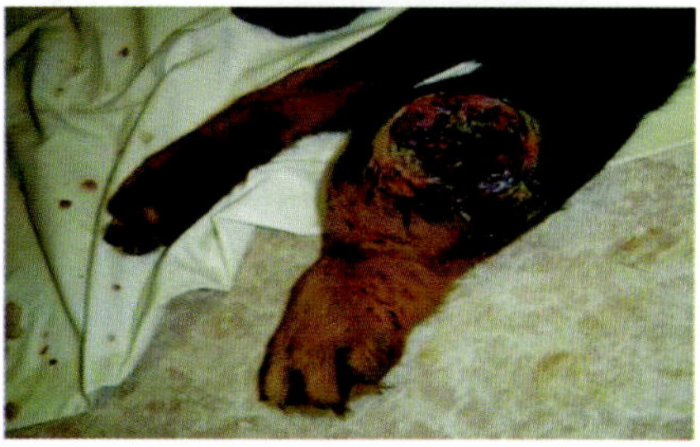

Fig.33. Ulcerating Wound

Evulsion/Avulsion wound: Here there is actual loss of tissue. E.g. Evulsion/Avulsion of horn or hoof. (fig.29).

Closed wounds: is a wound in which there is no break in the continuity of skin or mucous membrane but the underlying tissues are damaged to a varying degree. Eg., Contusion (fig.30), Bruise, Haematoma (fig.31).

Classification based on contamination of wound

1. Aseptic wound
2. Contaminated wound
3. Infected wound

1. Aseptic wound

Surgical wound made under aseptic condition when all the chances of contamination of wound is avoided. (fig.32)

2. Contaminated wound

Any wound other than aseptic wound. Infecting microorganisms will be present in fresh wound.

3. Infected /septic wound

Microorganisms invaded into the wound and multiplied in the wound causing the infection. Any wound after lag phase of 6-8 hrs is called as infected wounds.

Classification based on healing

1. Granulating wound.
2. Ulcerating wound.

1. Granulation wound

Granulation wound is one showing healing tissue inside the wound. Because of this wounds will appear red moist velvet appearance and will bleed easily.

2. Ulcerating wound

Which show no healing appear peal with an elevated fibrous around the wound. (fig.33)

Factors Affecting Wound Healing

1. Bacterial infection
2. Foreign bodies in wound-thorns, suture material, dead tissue.
3. Devitalisation of tissues-act as good source for bacterial growth.
4. Desiccation of tissues-due to prolonged exposure to air
5. Hematomas and serum collection-act as good sorce for growth of bacteria.
6. Inadequate blood supply-wide gap/dead space– healing affected
7. Presence of neoplastic tissue.
8. Lack of immobilisation-frequent movement-causes rupture of granulation tissue.
9. Chemical and mechanical trauma
10. Old age
11. Malnutrition—esp. protein deficiency
12. Vitamin K deficiency-necessary for formationof intercellular substance and maturation of collagen
13. Deficiency of other vitamins—vitamin D, A, B.
14. Surgical technique.
15. Tissue vascularity.
16. Mechanical stress.
17. Movement.
18. Extent of wound surface.
19. Odema and dehydration.
20. Local irradiation.
21. Wound infection.
22. Dehydration.

Symptoms of wound: Classified into three symptoms.

1. Local Symptoms
2. General symptoms,
3. Remote symptoms.

Local Symptoms

Hemorrhage, pain, gaping of wound lips and signs of tissue repair.

General symptoms: 2 types

A. Febrile disturbances: Extent of injury and severity/virulence of organ, there will be rise of temperature.

B. Toxaemic: enlargement of draining lymph glands, pain, fever (due to toxins absorbed from wound site).

Remote symptoms

Are those appear at places away from sites of wound, abscessation of bleeding lymph glands neuralgia, paralysis. Wound at axilla can damage brachial plexus and cause fore limb paralysis.

Treatment of wound

Contusion wound: Application of cold astringents, control immediate inflammation, e.g. Magnesium sulphate, acetic acid chalk piece.

Ulcerating wound

Which show no signs of healing. Appear pale with an elevated fibrous ring round the wound.

Haematoma

If small, no treatment is required, gets absorbed gradually. If large open, drain and treated just like open wounds. Aseptic wounds can be sutured.

Contaminated wound

Treatment includes 5 steps

1. Control bleeding.
2. Cleaning of wounds.
3. Control of infection.
4. Providing drainage.
5. Immobilization.

1. **Control of bleeding**: If fresh less bleeding will be there. If wound is extensive or larger blood vessel is involved, normal clotting mechanism does not happen. So various haemostatic will be applied. Apply local styptics. Alum, Tincture benzoin, Parenteral coagulants like vit k, Adrenochrome, Ligation can also be done if it is larger.
2. **Cleaning of wound:** Clip/shave the hairs around the wound, clean it, and scrub with antiseptic lotions to remove dirt and dead tissues, Common antiseptics are used. Perchloride of mercury 1 in 1000, Potassium permanganate solution 1:1000, Acriflavin 1:1000, Hypertonic saline solution 5-10% Povodine Iodine solution, Chlorhexidine solution.

   If volume of dead tissue is more can be sniffed off to the extent possible and can be separated till wound is clean. After wound edges are made clean we can think of suturing the edges if possible. Infected wound are left unsutured for the fear of accumulation of exudates and may require regular irrigation on daily/alternate days. Wound on feet can be treated with warm foot baths of 10% formalin.
3. **Control of infection:** Cover the wound with antiseptics ointment, powders or lotions. If there is any suspect of infection go for parental therapy. If wounds have started healing process, then avoid using strong antiseptics.
4. **Providing drainage**: Presence of exudates or discharges will delay wound healing. Drainage will be provided in such wounds especially when wound is deep. Enlarging wound opening keeping fenestrated tube from depths of wound or gauze pieces dipped in antiseptics can also be used or providing counter opening when fluid do not move against gravity. So counter openings are made at dependent portion region for facilitating gravity force to drain the wound.
5. **Immobilization of wound:** Excess movement of wound edges will delay wound healing. Excess granulation tissue protruding due to lack of immobilization is called 'Proud flesh or exuberant granulation'.

Immobilization is by

1. Suturing the wound edges
2. Apply bandage or adhesive tapes.
3. Apply splints.

Treatment of punctured wound

External opening has to be enlarged and punctured openings are cauterized with red hot shoe nail. If wounds are on hoof, hoof can be tarred with tarring knife. We can cut some part of wound so that wound become large, remove the dead tissue, then go for treatment with antiseptic foot bath (formalin 40%), antiseptics are used for treating wound. Strict course of antibiotics are used.

Avulsion of hoof or horn

1. Control of bleeding by styptics/tourniquet.
2. Wash and dress the region, remove clots adhering, clip nail.
3. Wound is bandaged, apply a moist antiseptic band, next day bandage is removed and dressed with oily dressing. This is repeated on every alternate day. After few days a growth of layer of horn takes place over the wound surface. Development of horn tissue takes months to get full growth.

Complications of wound healing

1. Heamorrhage.
2. Wound dehiscence.
3. Traumatic neuralgia.
4. Traumatic fever and septicaemia.
5. Traumatic emphysema.
6. Tetanus.
7. Haematoma or seroma.
8. Sinus.
9. Fistula.
10. Cellulitis

EN-BLOC DEBRIDMENT

Complete excision of wound without entering the wound. Indicated in wounds which are infected without signs of systemic infection. Done where there is sufficient tissue and no vital nerves, vessels or tendons.

Technique: Pack the wound with gauze and close edges over gauze. Excise the mass (as if a tumour) such that gauze is never expose. The advantage of this technique is that it removes all damaged and contaminated tissue.

□□□

ANESTHESIOLOGY

10

History

- In 1665 Physician Elsholz used a solution of opium to produce unconsciousness in a patient.
- In 1776 nitrous oxide was discovered by Joseph Priestly. (fig. 34)
- In 1821, Benjamin Brodie demonstrated the anesthetic properties of ether. (fig. 35)
- In 1824, Henry Hill Hickman experimented with carbon dioxide. He believed that anesthesia caused by nitrous oxide is because of CO_2 enhancing the rate and depth of breathing. (fig.36)
- In 1930's US dentist Horace Wells used nitrous oxide for tooth extraction. (fig.37)
- British veterinarians demonstrated the apparently successful use of Curare as a muscle relaxant in tetanus in 1835.
- Laughing gas properties were popular in the United States during the 1830's and about 1840 "ether frolics" became the similar attraction.
- Anesthesia pioneer Dr. Crawford W. Long was the first to use anesthesia during an operation, giving it to his friend before excising a cyst from his neck. He was the first to investigate ether anesthesia on animals in 1842. (fig.38)
- Thomas Morton on October 16, 1846 was the first person to demonstrate Ether anesthesia in Public at Massachusetts General Hospital. (fig.39)
- 1850's ice was used as a form of regional anesthesia for limb amputation.

- Plato was the first writer to use the term anesthesia, although not with specific reference to its induction: the latter honor goes to Oliver Wendall Holmes (1846), although the term was used during the 18th century to denote loss of sensation, as by freezing. (Fig.40)
- John Snow administered chloroform to Queen Victoria for the birth of Prince Leopold on 7th April 1853. She later wrote in her journal "Dr. Snow gave that blessed chloroform and the effect was soothing, quieting and delightful beyond measure". (fig.41)
- Ether spray discovered by Benjamin Richardson in 1867.
- 1897 August 16, German surgeon Dr. August Bier administered the first spinal anesthesia in animals. (Fig.42)
- Discovery of procaine in 1904 and its clinical application by Braun in 1905.
- With the employment of an ether-oil mixture and quinine, the technique was highly popular during the 1920's in obstetrics.
- Tribromethanol was introduced as a rectal anesthetic in 1927 and during the 1930's was widely used in Britain for cats before the barbiturates were discovered.
- George H. Dadd appears to have been the first veterinary practioner to use ether or chloroform for surgical anesthesia.
- Ernest H. Volwiler and Donalee L. Tabern, working for Abbott Laboratories, discovered Sodium thiopental in the early 1930s.

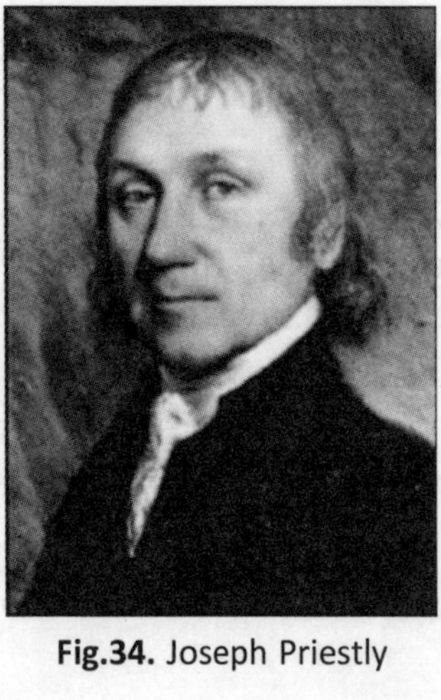

Fig.34. Joseph Priestly

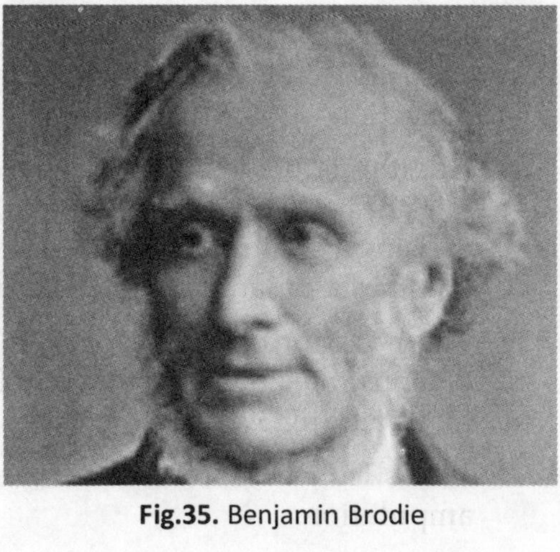

Fig.35. Benjamin Brodie

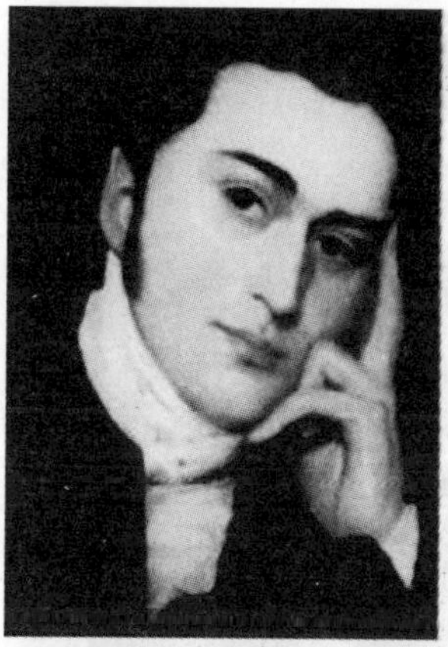

Fig.36.HenryHill Hickman

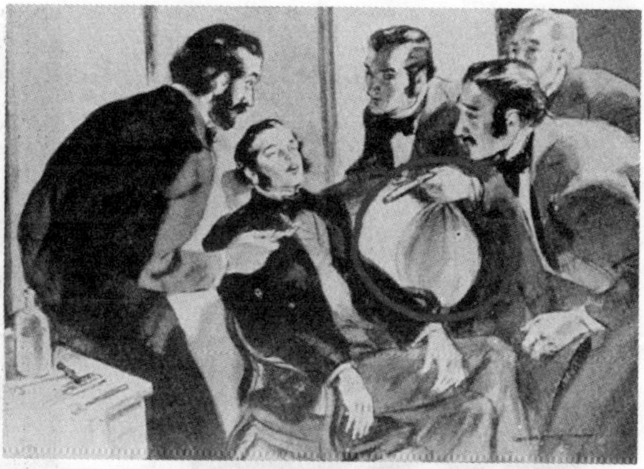

Fig.37. Use of Nitrous oxide for tooth extraction By Horace Wells

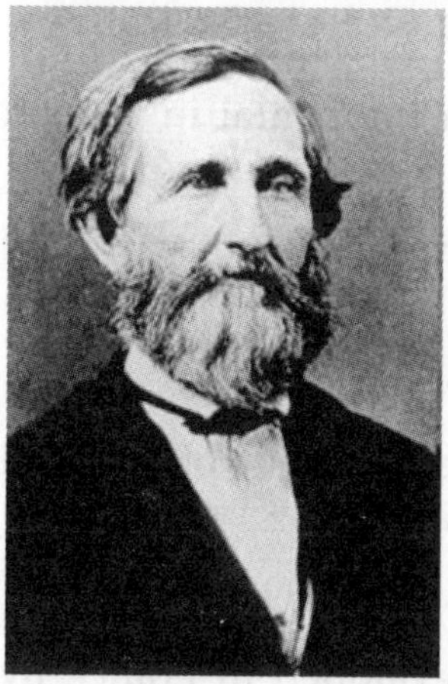

Fig.38. W.C.Wang

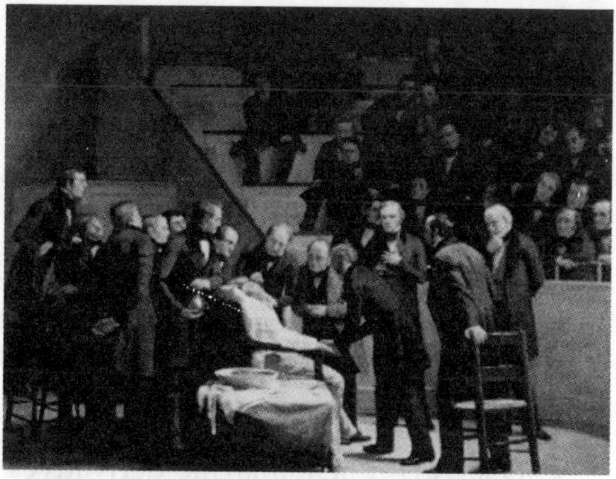

Fig.39. Thomas Morton demonstrate Ether anesthesia

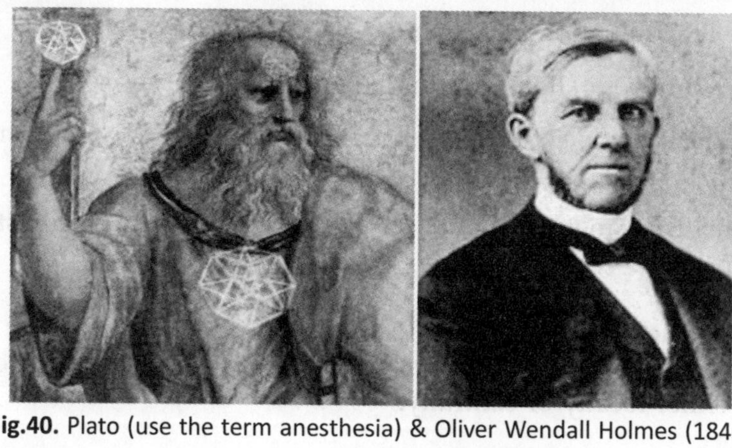

Fig.40. Plato (use the term anesthesia) & Oliver Wendall Holmes (1846)

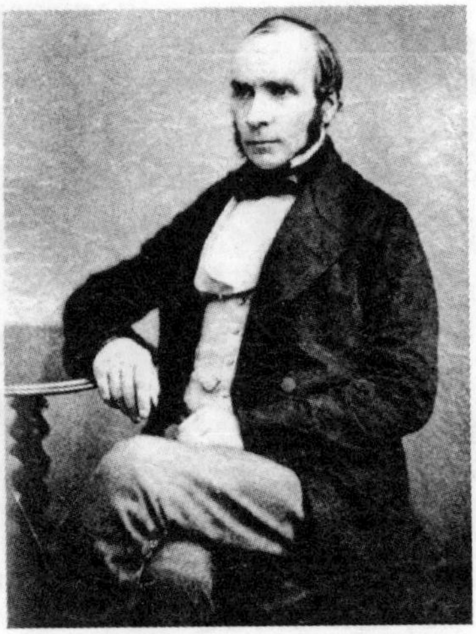

Fig.41. John Snow

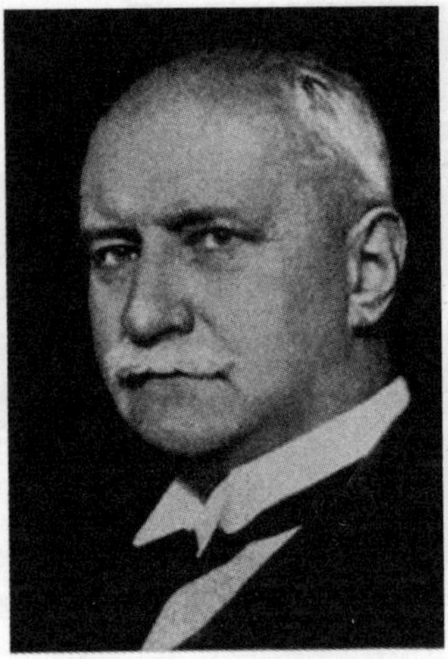

Fig .42. August Bier

- Dr. Ralph M. Waters first used Sodium thiopental in human beings on March 8, 1934.
- Cuille and Sendrail (1901) of France introduced sub-arachnoid anesthesia in Horses, Cattle and Dogs.
- Cathelin (1901) reported epidural analgesia in the Dog.
- Retzgen, Benesch and Brook reported the technique of epidural anesthesia in Large animal species in 1920s.
- 1940 A.D- I/V anesthesia in veterinary surgery was started.
- 1950 A.D- Phenothiazine derivatives developed in France by Charpantier.
- 1966 Evaluation of Enflurane in animals.
- 1970 Introduction of Ketamine in animal surgery.
- American Society of Veterinary Anesthesiology was formed in 1970.
- In 1975 American College of Veterinary Anesthesiologists was formed.

Anesthesia is used to denote loss of sensation to any part or whole of the body, produced by agents, which depress the activity of nervous tissue either locally or centrally.

Local anesthesia is a loss of sensation in a limited body area.

Regional anesthesia is a loss of sensation or insensibility in larger, but limited body area.

General anesthesia is complete unconsciousness.

Surgical anesthesia is a state of unconsciousness, where adequate muscular relaxation is produced to perform surgical operation painlessly.

Analgesia is a relief from pain

Tranquilization is a state of behavioral change in which the patient is relaxed but unconcerned of his surroundings.

Sedation is a state of mild degree central depression, where the patients is awake but calm.

Narcosis: is a state of deep sleep accompanied by analgesia

Hypnosis: is an artificially induced sleep and results from moderate depression of central nervous system.

Types of anesthesia

1. Local analgesia
    a. By surface application
    b. By intra- and subdermal infiltration. (fig.43)
    c. Field anesthesia: the blocking of an area by linear infiltration of its margins.
2. Regional anesthesia
    a. By perineural injection
    b. Spinal block
    i. Epidural injection (fig.44)
    ii. Intrathecal injection

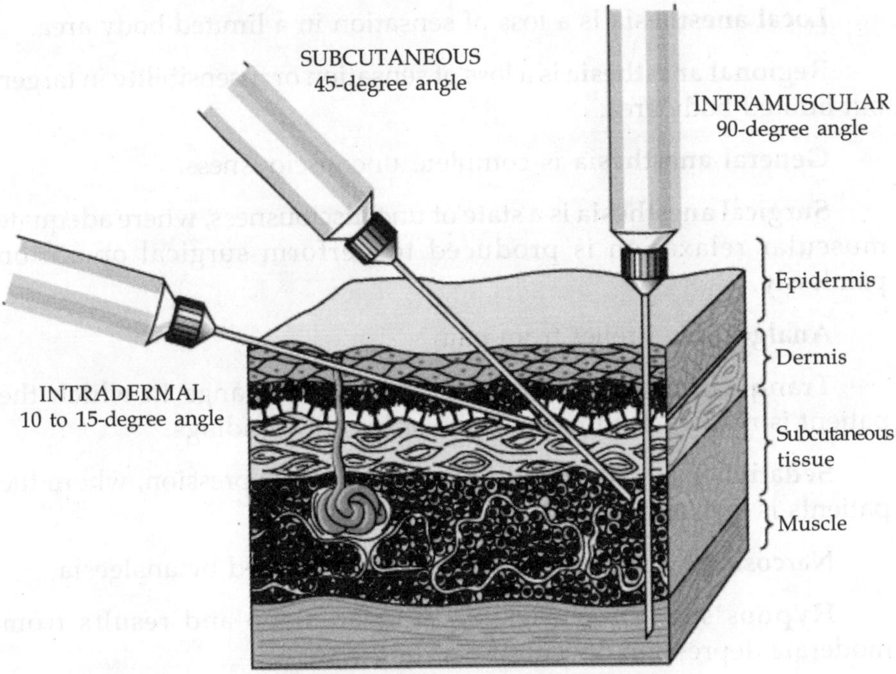

Fig.43. Intra- dermal infiltration

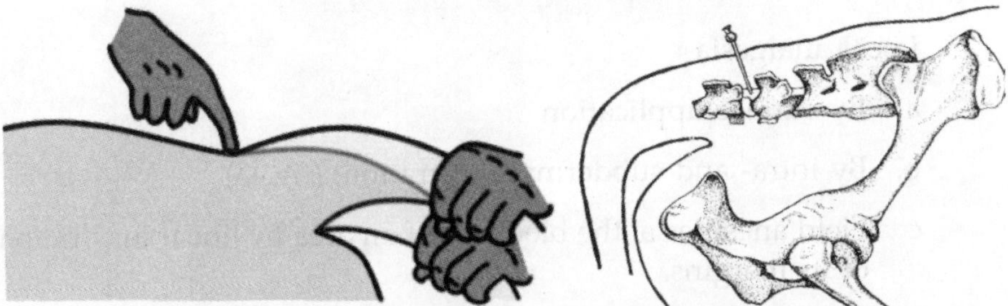

Fig.44. Caudal epidural injection in cattle

3. Sedation and norcosis
   a. In combination with local or regional analgesia.
   b. As an adjunct to general anesthesia
4. General anesthesia
   a. By inhalation
   b. By oral, rectal, intravenous or intraperitoneal administration of a non- volatile anesthetic
   c. By a combination of the two with or without premedication.

Selection of anesthetic agent depends upon

1. Time required performing a surgical procedure.
2. The metabolic rate of an animal; very young animal has low metabolism and limited muscular and adipose tissue and immature detoxification mechanism.
3. Age of the animal: aged animals are often poor anesthetic risk mainly due to possibility of presence of chronic heart, liver or kidney disease.
4. Breed: brachycephalic dogs having pendulous soft palate and restricted respiratory passages have difficulty in breathing.
5. Species difference: regional anesthesia is most desirable in cattle, buffaloes and goats since general anesthesia is complicated by hazards of ruminal tympany, regurgitation and aspiration.
6. Type of surgery / surgeon: barbiturates are contraindicated for caesarean section because of the respiratory depression of new born. General anesthesia with positive pressure ventilation are used for surgery of thorax or thoracic organs.
7. Physical state or health of animal.
8. Availability of equipment and personnel.

❑❑❑

11

Preanaesthetic Considerations and Preanaesthetics

Preanaesthestic drugs are used to prepare the patient for induction and contribute to the maintenance and smooth recovery from anesthesia. Specifically these drugs are chosen to;

1. Calm down the patient
2. Induce sedation
3. Provide analgesia and muscle relaxation
4. Decrease the airway secretion
5. Decrease the autonomic reflex responses
6. To decrease the fluid volume and acidity
7. To suppress or prevent vomition/regurgitation during anesthesia
8. Decrease anesthetic requirement and promotes smooth induction and recovery from anesthesia.

Drugs include

- Anticholinergics
- Tranquilizers
- Sedatives
- Opioids
- Opioid + tranquilizer combination (neurolept analgesics).

Anticholinergics

1. Atropine sulfate

It blocks the Ach at postganglionic termination of cholinergic fibers autonomic nervous system it decreases the oral, pharyngeal, respiratory tract secretions and dilates the bronchi. Atropine sulfate increases both anatomical and physiological dead space & accentuate the postoperative hypoxemia. Motor and secretory activity in the GIT is decreased and vagal influence on the heart is suppressed. In therapeutic doses, it alters the arterial blood pressure minimally. It blocks the cholinergic fibers of short ciliary nerve and relaxes the sphincter muscle of iris, dilates the pupil. Doesn't dilate the pupil of the birds because iris is made of striated muscle.

Atropine sulfate decreases the tear formation in awake anaesthetized dogs. It is contraindicated in animals with preexisting tachycardia.

Dosage

Cattle: 0.04-0.06 mg /kg it doesn't decrease the saliva production but make the saliva more viscid.

Swine: 0.06-0.08 mg/kg

Dog: 0.04 mg/kg If 0.5 mg/kg through i/v causes excitement and decreases thiopentone requirement by 25% and doubles the duration of anesthesia in dogs. Atropine sulfate when given i/v at 0.044 mg/kg. Intravenous to dogs recovering from thiopentone anesthesia is reinduced and duration is longer

Ponies: i/v 0.44 mg and 0.176mg/kg stops the intestinal motility and colic respectively. So contraindicated.

2. Glycopyrolate : (Robinal ^{R})

It is a Quaternaryammonium compounds, anticholinergic drug has a prolonged antisialogouge effect, has no effect on vision and Cardiovascular system. Glycopyrolate is more potent than Atropine sulfate. Glycopyrrolate system seems to be less likely than Atropine to produce sinus tachycardia. It does not penetrate the CNS because of its difficulty in crossing the blood-brain barrier. It is also less likely than Atropine to cross the placental barrier, indicating that it is a selective peripheral anticholinergic agent.

Dog: 0.011mg/kg

Tranzuilizers

Primarily used to relieve anxiety. May be used to quiten the patient for physical examination & transport to prevent chewing bandages & splints, as an anti emetic especially for prevention of "Car sickness" or "Motion sickness".

When tranquilizers are given as preanesthetics induction & motion sickiness is easy and dose is reduced & incidence of vomition is reduced, recovery from anesthesia is smooth & free from struggling & vocalization.

3 groups: 1.Phenothiazines 2. Butyrophenones 3. Benzodiazepam

1. Phenothiazines

Decreases the epinephrine induced disarrythmias. Produce sedation and reduce the dose of drugs needed for general anesthesia, but also cause moderate hypotension and hypothermia.

Promethazine HCI : (Phenargon R)

Used often as an antihistaminic in veterinary practice & can also cause sedative effect.

Chlorpromazine Hcl: (Largactil R, TranchlorR)

Used for tranquilization & antiemetic activity. It is a powerful CNS depressant with moderate antiemetic activity.

In cattle: since it produces profound CNS depression it is strictly given I/m route only

In horses: contraindicated because it causes excitement.

Dogs & cats: 0.5-1 mg/kg.i/m,i/v route. Oral dose 1-2 mg/kg.

In cattle, pig, sheep, and goat: 1 mg/kg, only i/m route.

Promazine Hcl : (sparine R)

Action is similar to largactil once drug of choice in horses before acepromazine was introduced.

Dog & cats: 0.5-1 mg/kg i/m, i/v.

Horses: 0.5 mg/kg. I/v.

Acetylpromazine: (Acepromazine [R]) (ACP)

Very effective preanaesthetic can be administered orally, s/c, i/m, or i/v route. Apart from tranquilization effect has a spasmolytic activity on smooth muscle, so also used to treat colic in horses.

Dogs: 0.03 – 0.01 mg/kg total dose shouldn't exceed 3 mg/kg

Cats: 0.03 -0.1 mg/kg

Cattle, sheep, and pig: 0.025-0.1 mg/kg i/m. Horses: 0.02-0.05 mg/kg.

Triflupromazine Hcl: (siquil [R])

A powerful CNS depressant has antiemetic property also. However Acepromazine & xylazine is most frequently used in equines & bovines.

Dogs & cats: 1-2 mg/kg i/m.

0.5-1 mg/kg i/v.

Cattle: 10-20 mg/kg i/v.

Powerful respiratory depressant & overdosage produces respiratory arrest.

Trimeprazine Hcl: (vallergon [R])

Good CNS depressant like sparin & largactil has specific antipruritic activity used in small animal dermatological affections as an antipruritic.

2. Butyrophenones

Have similar effects as phenothiazines, but are more potent and cause less hypotension.

Droperidol

A drug with powerful tranquilization effect and antiemetic action also. However in dogs causes retching. Not used in veterinary practice but used with fentanyl (narcotic) as a neurolept analgesic drug as innovarvet [R].

3. Benzodiazepines

Bring about good sedation and tranquilization with muscle relaxation, muscle relaxation is at CNS level and because of this they are also used to control seizures and spasms.

a) Diazepam: Valium®, Calmpose®

When administered brings about tranquilization and also muscle relaxation. Solution is irritant and so it is given deep I/M injection or I/V. Clinical dose does not alter CNS function.

Dogs and Cats: 0.1-0.5 mg/Kg I/V

0.3-1.0 mg/kg I/M

Horses; 0.05-0.2mg/Kg I/V

Pig, Sheep and Cattle 0.5-1 mg/ kg I/M

Chicken and Turkey 5-10 mg/Kg I/M.

b) Zolazepam: Telazole®

Powerful benzodiazepine used in combination with teletamine (good for felines).

c) Midazolam

Water soluble benzodiazepine, used in small animals at 0.1-0.2 mg/Kg.

4. Alpha-2-Adrenergic Agonists (xylazine, detomidine, medetomidine)

i) Xylazine (Rompun) is a sedative and analgesic that acts as Central Nervous System depressant and induces muscle relaxation by inhibiting the transmission of impulses in the Central nervous system. Its major use in laboratory animal anesthesia is in combination with ketamine to produce surgical anesthesia.

This combination has been used in dogs, cats, NHP, large farm animals and wild animals. It causes respiratory depression and a bradycardia which may progress to heart block. It also increases the susceptibility of the myocardium to circulating catecholamines during halothane anesthesia. Vomiting may occur in dogs and cats, and gas accumulation due to gastrointestinal atony (lack of normal tone or strength) may be a problem in both large dogs and ruminants. Xylazine produces profound physiological changes and its safe use requires knowledge of these effects which are often species specific. Yohimbine and 4-aminopyridine reverse most of the effects of xylazine without relapse in many species, with the exception of NHP. (Non human Trimates).

OPIOIDS (Narcotic analgesics)

Most powerful systemic analgesics known. Used in varieties of ways :

- Relief of post operative pain
- Relief of pre operative pain
- Used as Neurolept analgesics.

Narcotic analgesics stimulate and depress CNS; overall affect depends on species of animal and the dose rate of administration.

The action due to depression of CNS includes :

1. Analgesia
2. Respiratory depression
3. Sedation and hypnosis
4. Depression of cough reflexes

Action due to stimulation of CNS includes :

1. General excitement and convulsions
2. Nausea and vomiting
3. Euphoria.

1. Morphine

An alkaloid extracted from ***Papaver somniferum***, as the alkaloid itself, is insoluble in water it is used as one of its soluble salts like sulphates or hydrochlorides. First isolated by Suturner in 1803. The word morphine is given after the Greek god of dreams- Morpheus. It is powerful naturally occurring sedative and analgesic. The therapeutic doses have no effect on CNS and respiratory system.

Dogs- Profound analgesia and sedation. Pupil become pin pointed because of excitation of nucleus of occulomotar nerve.

Cat- Maniacal excitement therefore contraindicated.

Horses, cattle and pigs- Effects are unreliable and sometimes bring about delirium and excitement.

Morphine crosses placental barrier and therefore is contraindicated in Caesarian, however it does not alter the uterine contraction during parturition.

Horses and cattle: Upto 60 mg as total dose

Dogs: Upto 10mg total

Pigs: Upto 20mg total

Synthetic morphine - Buprenorphine (Dog 0.02 mg/Kg I/M or I/V)

2. Pathedine HCL or Meperidine

Potent CNS depressant used as and for post operative analgesia. Analgesic effect is 1/10th that of morphine. Therapeutic doses do not change CNS system and muscular activity.

Dogs 2.5-6.5 mg/ kg as pre anesthetic

5-10 mg/Kg for post operative analgesic.

3. Fentanyl : Sublimaze ®, Phentanyl®

Potent narcotic analgesic, 250 times more potent than morphine on mg to mg basis. Rapid onset of action with I/M that is in 5 minutes and reaches the peak in 30 minutes and thereafter diminishes. Bradycardia is observed due to vagal tone and this can be minimized by prior Atropinisation. As such fentanyl is not used in veterinary practice but used as neurolept analgesia with droperidol.

Fentanyl +droperidol gives Innovarvet dose of which is 1ml /10 Kg body weight I/M or 1ml / 30 Kg body weight I/ V.

Sedation and analgesia sets in 3-4 minutes and recommended for minor surgical procedures along with local anesthesia.

When Innovar vet is used as pre anesthetic medicant with gaseous anesthesia the dose is 1/4th to 1/2 the original dose.

Innovar vet is extensively used in primates :

Rhesus monkey	0.05 ml/kg B.W
Large primates	1 ml/kg B.W

Pentazocin Hcl: Fortwin ®

Potent analgesic in canines

Onset of action	½ hour
Duration	4-5 hour
Dosage	0.5 mg/kg B.W

4. Etorphine M 99

Most powerful narcotic analgesic available. 0.5 mg of etorphine has a narcotic effect for 500 kg. Extensively used for wild animals especially rogue elephants (antidote is Revivone ® or naloxone) used by darting. Powerful CNS depressant and bring about profound bradycardia and respiratory depression. Once the animal is restrained the effect should be reversed by diprenorphine (M55 ® revivon ®) by volume to volume basis dose. 1 ml of etorphine = 1 ml revivon or 0.272 mg/kg I/v naloxone: can also be used as an antidote at 0.6 -0.8 mg/kg.

Etorphine-wear glass while handling because it is absorbed through intact skin.

Butorphenol : Torbugesic ®

Equine use. It is synthetic morphine 3 x morphine

Dogs: 0.1 0.3 mg/kg B.W

Horses: 0.1 -0.4 mg/kg

□□□

12

Local Analgesia /Anaesthesia

Definition: Loss of sensation in a limited body area.

Classification of Local Analgesia

1. Surface analgesia
   a. Skin
   b. Mucus membrane
2. Infiltrate analgesia
   a. 'L' block (fig.45)
   b. 'T' block
   c. Diamond block (fig.46)
   d. Field block
3. Regional analgesia
   a. Spinal/Epidural anesthesia
      i. Anterior epidural
      ii. Posterior epidural
   b. Perineural analgesia
      i. Paravertebral
      ii. Specific nerve blocks.

Mechanism of Action

Local anesthetics they mainly act by blocking the conduction in peripheral nerves. They mainly inhibit sodium influx through voltage gated sodium channels. Local anesthetic binds rapidly open sodium channels. So it becomes a state dependent blockage.

When local anesthesia is infiltrated around the nerve. Loss of function occurs first in unmyelinated then in smaller myelinated, then in larger myelinated. Because myelin is impervious to anesthetic, increased number of nodes action will be rapid.

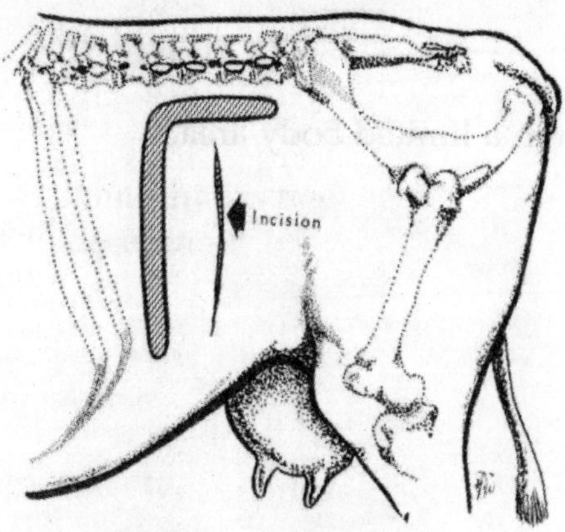

Fig.45. Inverted L Block

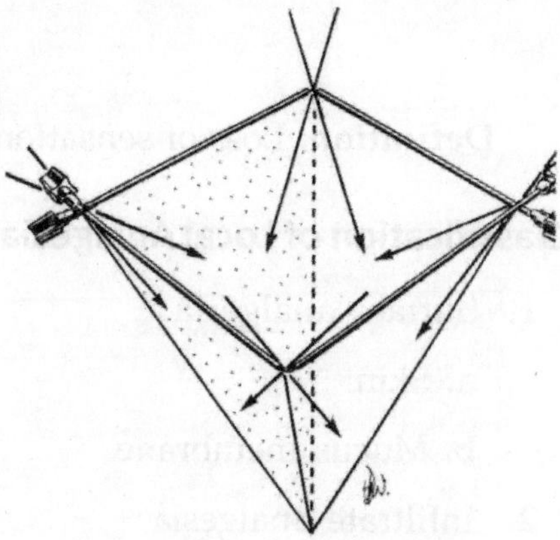

Fig.46. Diamond Block

Agents

Two types: 1. Amino amide 2. Amino esters

1. **Amino amides**
   - Bupivacaine
   - Levobupivacaine
   - Lidocaine
   - Mepivacaine
   - Prilocaine
   - Ropivacaine
   - Combinations of lidocaine and prilocaine

2. Amino esters

- Benzocaine
- Chloroprocaine
- Cocaine
- Procaine

Lidocaine (xylocaine) – 1940 Modern local anesthetic widely used anesthetic even today in America.

Agents

Cocaine

Action: Paralysis of sensory nerve endings also has analgesic and vasoconstrictor effect.

Doses: Subcutaneous infiltration

Horses : 780 mg Small Dogs: 45 mg

Large dogs : 120 mg Cats: 15 mg

4% solution – eye instillation

10 to 20% - Nasal and laryngeal.

Procaine

- Less toxic than cocaine
- General infiltration skin and gums – dogs and cats – 2%.
- Epidural – 1 to 2.5% concentration.
- Perineural injection – 4 to 5% - horses and cattle.
- Onset – 5 to 10mmts – persists for an hour.

Tutocaine

More potent then procaine.

Amethocaine HCl

Used for desensitization of mucus membrane.

1% solution – installation eye.

2% solution – pharynx, larynx, nasal mucus membrane.

Propoxycaine

Dental anesthesia – 2% procaine with 0.4% popoxycaine.

Cinchocaine

Used for surface and spinal analgesia.

Lingocaine HCl

Available as lidocaine/xylocaine/xylotox has more penetration power as compared to others. Causes less tissue damage/irritation, used on mucus membrane/cornea – 4% solution. Over dose causes drowsiness, twitching, respiratory depression, convulsion and hypotension.

Dosage - Infiltration

Horses and cattle: 6gm / 300ml of 2% solution

Dogs: 0.6g/30ml of 2% solution

Mepivocaine HCl

Dogs – 29 mg/kg (dosage)

Bupivocaine HCl (Marcain)

Available along with adrenaline, more potent than lignocaine.

Techniques / Methods

I. **Surface analgesia** – agents which cause freezing of superficial skin. Used for passage of stomach tube in dogs. Used for intrasynovial analgesia examination of glans penis/vulva. On intact skin anesthesia can be produced by ether spray/ethyl chloride/carbonic acid. The action is within 20 to 30 seconds. Mucus membrane – anesthesia can be produced by using 4% lignocaine HCl in the form of Gel / aqueous solution for ointment.

II. **Infiltration analgesia** – nerve endings are affected at the actual site of operation. Types :

Field block: Making walls of analgesia enclosing the operation field. Eg. Inverted block 'L' block used for ruminotomy.

Ring block: Used for amputation of digits. Teats operation.

Diamond block: Used for tumor exicision, LN biopsy.

'T' block: Anesthesia is infiltrated in the shape of 'T'.

III. **Regional Anesthesia** - refers to loss of sensation in a larger area though a limited body area.

a. **Intravenous regional analgesia** - Beir - 1908. Anesthetic solution is injected to superficial vein below the tourniquet.

1. **Spinal or Epidural anesthesia** - Anatomical considerations - Spinal cord is that portion of brain lodged in the spinal canal. Spinal cord opens cranially at IV ventricle of brain. Caudally terminates forming cone like structure - conus medullaries a bundle of nerves arise from the conus modularizes - cauda equine resembles the tail of horse.

   Spinal cord is covered by three layers of meninges: (1) Duramater, (2) Arachinoid (3) Piamater.

Spinal cord has two enlargements i,e Posterior cervical region and posterior lumbar region. In each vertebral segment canal has lateral opening between the vertebral arches i.e., IVF through which spinal nerves comes out.

Two types of spinal anesthesia :

1. Epidural anesthesia
2. Subarachinoid anesthesia

A. **Epidural Anesthesia**

Local anesthetic injected in spinal cord above the duramater spread of anesthesia depends on the concentration and quantity of solution used. Two types of epidural anesthesia : (a) Anterior/high and (b) Posterior/low.

Posterior Block: Motor control of hind limb is intact.

Anotomical regions affected - anus, vulva, perineum, posterior aspect of thigh, relaxation of anal sphincter and dialatation of vagina.

Dosage - 2% procaine HCl 2% lignocaine HCl

Heifer - 5ml

Medium sized - 10ml

Large - 15ml

Onset of action takes 1 to 1 ½ min. peak will be there at 15-20 mints. lasts for one hour.

OX: Saccroccocygeal space is preferred because space is larger, anesthetic solution spreads easily, 8-10ml of 2% lignocaine HCl is injected it completely blocks the sensory nerves. The site is located by elevating and lowering the tail and palpating depression between the last sacral and first coccygeal or between first and second coccygeal vertebra. Ten cm long 18G needle is inserted at a median plane at 10-15° to the vertical.

Sheep and Goat: Cranial epidural block performed at lumbosacral space to desensitize the abdominal region.

Dog: Lumbosacral space is preferred. Indicated when animals are in shock and also when animals are aged where the use of other analgesic/anesthetic is contraindicated.

Technique: Spinal needle is placed perpendicular to skin surface at midline of lumboracral space, palpated half way between dorsoiliac-wings caudal to spinous process of 7th lumbar vertebra. Needle is inserted ventrally 2% lidocaine used at 1ml/10lb body weight.

B. Anterior block

Motor influence of hind is affected ranging from partial paralysis to complete paralysis lose of sensation seen in croup, inguinal regions, prepace, scrotum, hind limbs, mammary glands, flank, abdominal to the umballicus. Duration will be there for 2hrs. Inco-ordination continuous upto 3-4hrs.

Dosage Table. Anterior block (2% procaine solution)

	Embryotomoy	Amputation of digit, udder
Small sized adult	40ml	100ml
Medium sized	75	120
Large sized	100	150

Lumbar Segmental Epidural Analgesia

Provides broad belt analgesia encircling abdomen, involving parietal peritoneum. Develop within 10 min. and persists for 3hrs.

Agents: 2% tutocaine (10-15ml), 4% procaine HCl (10ml) 3% lignocaine HCl - heifer 6ml, adults-10ml.

Technique: Arthur's technique - 1.5cm behind anterior edge of second transverse process. Spinal needle directed downwards and inwards at an angle of 10 to 13° vertical. For a distance of 7.5 cm at which needle entered the neural canal, it is deposited.

Sheep: Site is located by palpation on each side on the anterior of ilium. Line joining these crosses the spinous process of last lumbar vertebra, needle is injected behind this. The area is thoroughly cleaned and disinfected before injection.

Agent: Lignocaine HCl (1 to 5%) + adrehaline. 1:100,000 dose - 8 to 10 ml effect will be there for 2 hrs.

Subarachinoid: Sheep used only when durameter is accidentally punctured.

Pigs: Lumbar epidural analgesia. Used to densentize the scrotum, testes, spermatic cord. 2% procaine 10ml is used along with adrenaline.

IV. **Perineural Injection**

A. NERVE BLOCKS-HEAD

OX

1. **Retrobulbar Nerve Block**: Blocks the nerves to ocular muscles producing paralysis of eye ball. (fig.47)

   Tech: 10-15ml of 2% lignocaine is used. Needle is inserted behind the middle of supraorbital process and pushed towards the last premolar of opposite side.

2. **Cornual Nerve Block**: Blocks the cornual nerves - bronch of lacrimal - ophthalmic - trigeminal nerve (CLOT). (fig.48)

   Tech: Needle is inserted to base of horn, lateral to palpable temporal ridge of frontal bone. 5-10ml of 2% lignocaine HCl is injected subcutaneously.

   Goat: Cornual branch of intratrochlear nerve and lacrimal nerve. Both blocked simuntaneously.

Equines

1. Auriculopalpebral nerve block (fig. 49)

   Indications: Examination and treatment of eye and ocular surgeries.

   Technique: Performed dorsal to zygomatic arch. Superficially inject 5ml of 2% lidocaine in a fan shaped manner.

2. Mental nerve block

   Indications: Analgesia of lower lip.

   Site: Lateral border of mental foramen on posterior border of mandible.

3. **Mandibular nerve block Indications**: Surgeries of lower jaw, teeth, alveoli. Performed medial aspect of mandible.

4. **Infraorbital never block**

   Indications: Upper lip, nose, cheek, medial canthus of eye.

   Site: Half distance from 2.5cm dorsal between nosomaxillary notch and rostral facial crest.

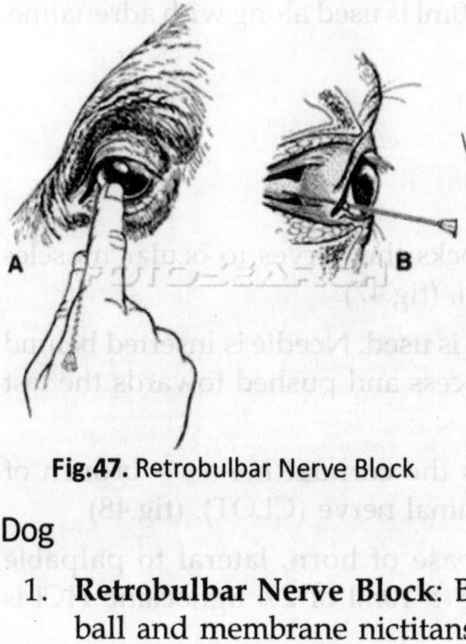

Fig.47. Retrobulbar Nerve Block

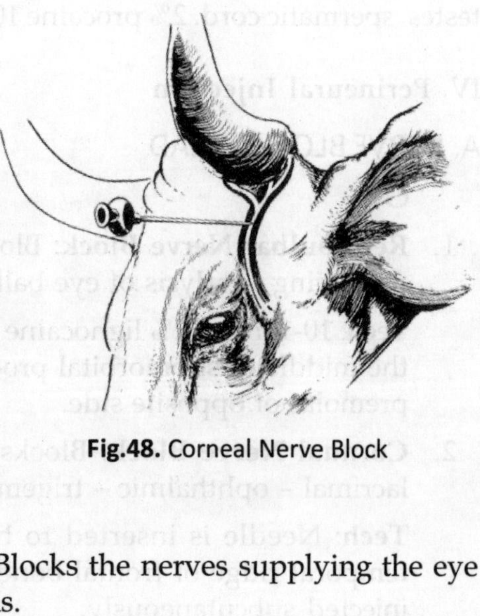

Fig.48. Corneal Nerve Block

Dog

1. **Retrobulbar Nerve Block**: Blocks the nerves supplying the eye ball and membrane nictitans.

   Tech: Curved needle is inserted through lateral canthus of eye 3-5ml of lidocaine solution is injected.

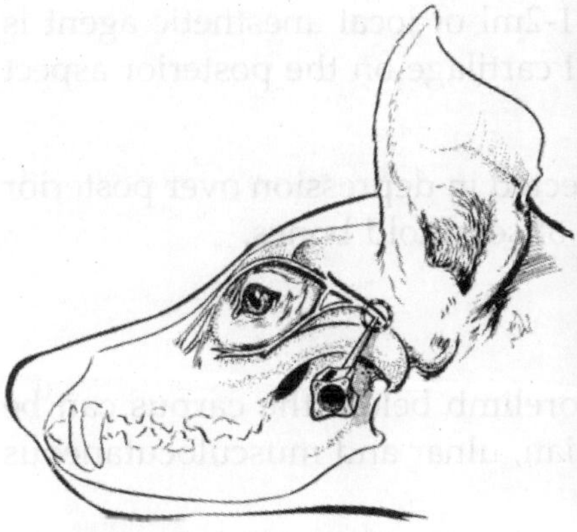

Fig.49. Retrobulbar Nerve Block

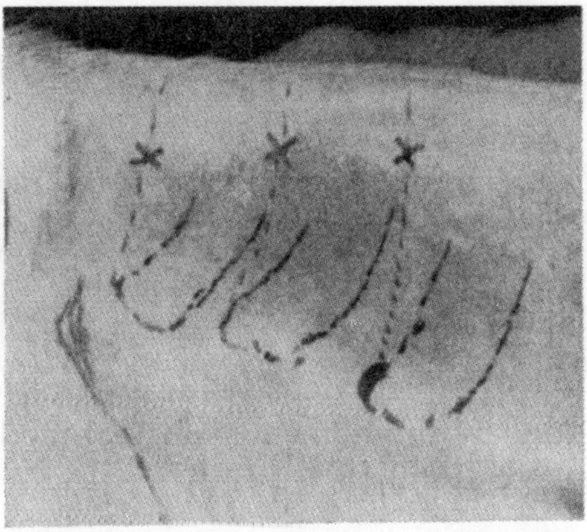

Fig.50. Site of paravertebral nerve block

2. **Auriculopalpabral Block**: Blocks motor innervation to the orbicularies occuli muscle.

   Tech: Needle is inserted subfacially over mid point of posterior third of zygomatic arch above its dorsal border.

3. **Supraorbital Nerve Block**: Used for upper eye lid operations forehead wound, trephining of frontal sinus.

   Tech: Needle is inserted midway across supraorbital process vertical line running upwards from medial angle of eye.

Nerve Blocks of Limb

Fore Limb

1. **Radial Nerve Block**: Blocked as it spirally moves around the humerus from medial to lateral surface midway between the olecranon and acromion process between long and lateral head of triceps. Supplies dorsal aspect of forearm and manus.
2. **Medial Nerve Block**: Sensory nerve supplying medial and dorsal surface of digit. Needle is inserted from cranial to medial epicondyle of humerus.
3. **Ulnar Nerve Block**: Performed hand breadth above the accessory carpal bone in the depression between ulnaries lateralies and flexor carpi ulnaries. 5-8ml anesthetic agent is injected.
4. **Musculocutaneous Nerve Block**: 5-10ml of anesthetic solution is injected subcutaneously on anteriomedial aspect of middle of forearm.

5. **Palmar Digital Nerve Block**: 1-2ml of local anesthetic agent is deposited at the level of lateral cartilage on the posterior aspect of 2nd phalanx.

6. **Digital Nerve Block**: 2-4ml injected in depression over posterior end of 1st phalanx/at the base of sesamoid bones.

Horse

Complete densensitization of forelimb below the carpus can be done by simultaneous block of median, ulnar and musculocutaneous nerve (10ml).

Hind Limb

1. **Peroneal Nerve Block**: Blocked behind the posterior edge of lateral condyle of tibia as it dips between the muscle bellys of extentors (6-12ml).
2. **Tibial Nerve Block**: Performed a hand spread above the hock, infront of tendoachilies on medial aspect between gastrocnemius tendon and flexor hellicus longus.

Horse

Plantar Block

1. **High Plantar Injection**: 2% lignocaine HCl, 2.5 to 7.5ml is injected 5 to 7cm above the fetlock joint subcutaneously.

2. **Low Plantar Injection**: Performed midway between the fetlock joint and coronet. 2-4ml solution is injected.

B. PARAVERTEBRAL ANAESTHESIA

The dorsal and ventral branches of T_{13}, L_1, L_2, L_3 are blocked.

Techniques

1. **Forguhorson's Tech**: Locate the last rib, then transverse process of posterior border T_{13} about 5 inches away from spinous process needle is passed vertically. For upper flank surgery T_{13}, L_1, L_2 and lower flank T_{13}, L_1, L_2, L_3 nerves are blocked. (fig.50)

2. **Magdas Method**: The skin is clipped and disinfected around the 1st, 2nd, 3rd, 4th lumbar transverse process 10ml of local analgesic solution is injected beneath each transverse process towards midline. This is more safer method.

Pudic Block (Internal Pudendal Block)

Brings about the exposure of bull's penis without causing locomotor impairment.

Tech: Nerve is located by rectal palpation at cranial angle of ischiatic arch by left hand by right hand inject the solution using 14 gauge and 12" long needle. 30ml of lignocaine is deposited around the nerve. Onset is by about 15-30 minutes lasts for 60 minutes.

Horse

Analgesia for castration can be produced using 2% lignocaine HCl/ 5% procaine HCl. 5ml is injected beneath the skin another 5ml injected to part of testis to desensitize the spermatic cord.

Dog

Paravertebral block-produced by last three thoracic and first four lumbar nerve block produces relaxation of abdominal muscles, so used in conjunction with light general anesthesia.

Complications and Management

The effect of local anesthetics not specific for signal conduction in peripheral nerves therefore conduction of electrical impulses follows similar mechanism in CNS and Heart.

1. **Central Nervous System**

   At lower concentrations cause cerebral excitation which may lead to convulsions. At higher concentrations lead to coma, respiratory arrest death (spinal anesthesia).

2. **Cardiovascular System** Cause atrioventricular block because of overdose can be treated using intravenous lipid emulsion (intralipid).

3. **Hypersensitivity / Allergy**

   Attributed to preservatives added to local anesthetic solution can be treated using adrenaline 1:1000 S/C injection, corticosteriods, antihistamines can also be used.

4. **Methemoglobinemia**

   Prilocaine metabolites induces this condition as it interferes with oxygen transport this side effect is potentially life threatening.

5. **Meningitis, post-operative malaise, paralysis** – due to damages to nerves.

6. **Toxicity** – cocaine when injected causes motor excitation.

7. **Fractures** – After nerve blocks of limb and also in the epidural anesthesia due to inco-ordination of the movement.

8. **Hypotension:** one of the common problems with local anaesthetic, characterized by small pulse, rapid, shallow respirations can be counteracted by I/V or I/M injections of vasopressors. Ex: metaraminol bitartarate (Aramine)-I/V-20mg. action within 1-3 minutes lasts for 25 to 30 minutes. It increases the myocardial contractions and peripheral resistance.

   Methoxamine HCl – I/V 30 to 60mg acts for 1hr.

□□□

13

General Anesthesia (Barbiturates and Dissociative Agents)

State of unconsciousness produced by a process of controlled, reversible intoxication of central nervous system, in which there is, lowered sensitivity to stimuli from the environment and a diminished motor response to such stimuli.

Anesthetic agents

Substance which produces both loss of consciousness and an absence of motor response to noxious stimuli in a controllable manner.

Routes of administration

1. Intra venous
2. Intra Muscular
3. Inhalation
4. Per Oral
5. Intra peritoneal
6. Subcutaneous
7. Per rectal
8. Epidural
9. Spinal

STAGES OF GENERAL ANESTHESIA

There are **4** stages:

Stage 1- stage of voluntary excitement or induction stage

Stage 2- stage of involuntary excitement

Stage 3- stage of anesthesia

Plane1- light plane

Plane 2- moderate plane

Plane 3- deep plane

Stage 4- stage of bulbar paralysis (over dosage stage)

Stage 1

Animal is conscious and it makes forcible efforts to avoid being anesthetized, during this stage breath holding may occur due to fear and apprehension, all body parameters are increased, pupils get dialated, vomition and defication may be seen.

Stage 2

On entering this stage animal loses its consciousness and reflex responses to stimuli, get exaggerated, movement of legs become violent and requires restraint at this stage, respiration is irregular, and oropharyngeal reflexes are still present. These disappears as the animal enters the next stage, in this stage dogs remain whimper or howl, cats may scream and horses may neigh.

Stage 3

Plane1: Regular anatomical breathing cessation of all limb movement, in large animals nystagmus occurs and finally the eye gets fixed at the centre indicating entry into the next phase. conjunctival, corneal and palpebral reflexes are still present, pedal reflex is brisk, in this stage the diagnostic investigation, minor surgical procedures like opening of abscess, can be performed.

Plane2: Little changes are noticed in dogs, eye ball takes ventromedial deviation, more muscular relaxation and pedal reflexes become sluggish, this plane is adequate for all surgeries except for intra abdominal surgeries.

Plane3: Anatomic regular breathing, respiratory rate is slightly buried and shallow, pause between inspiration and expiration, in dog eye ball return back to the centre, pupil are pin pointed, pedal reflexes are totally absent.

Stage 4

Paralysis of intercostal muscle occurs and diaphragm continues to work, during inspiration diaphragm contracts and causes relaxed abdominal wall to bulge called as "chynestoke respiration", pupils start dilating because of ciliary muscle paralysis (last muscle to relax in the body), eyeball become dry, cornea become wrinkled called as "fish eye", if there is over dosage, it causes hypo ventilation and leads to hypoxia, supplement oxygen and specific antidote can be given, resuscitation of lungs by artificial ventilation. Give respiratory analeptics like doxopram and nikethemide to overcome the condition.

TYPES

Intravenous Anesthesia

Inhalational Anesthesia

Barbiturates

Differ from tranquillizers and opioids in that increasing the dose progressively increases the depth of depression until a state of general anesthesia are reached. They are poor analgesics. Their primary use is in the induction and/or maintenance of general anesthesia. Barbiturates are potent respiratory depressants and their effects on the cardiovascular system are variable. At intermediate dosages, excitement is sometimes induced.

The barbiturates are grouped according to duration of action into long acting (e.g., phenobarbital), short- or intermediate-acting (e.g., pentobarbital) and ultrashort-acting (e.g., thiopental, thiamylal, and methohexital), the short- and ultra short-acting drugs are commonly used for anesthesia. Anesthetic duration varies widely with species; however, in general, short/intermediate barbiturates produce approximately 2-3 hours of anesthesia and ultrashort barbiturates range from 10 to 20 minutes.

Variation in dose response and duration of effect of barbiturates is extreme within and between species. The following are examples of the variation found with pentobarbital (intermediate) anesthesia:

i) Cats frequently having a considerably prolonged sleeping time.

ii) Mice on hardwood bedding take almost twice as long to recover as mice on softwood bedding, and male mice sleep longer than female mice.

iii) The anesthesia produced in adult horses and cattle is of relatively short duration; however, the recovery period is long and difficult.

Whenever possible, barbiturates should be administered intravenously, slowly, to effect. Administration by other routes is far less satisfactory, as dosage is more difficult to judge and the anesthetic effects are less predictable. Any of the barbiturates can cause skin sloughing if perivascular injection accidentally occurs.

Although barbiturates are commonly used, they are often poor choices for general anesthesia due to poor analgesia, profound cardiovascular effects, high mortality and numerous external factors that can affect dose response and sleeping time. Adequate anesthesia can be obtained by combining a barbiturate with a tranquillizer, sedative or an opioid.

Thiopentone sodium: A thio analogue of pentobarbital sodium. Reconstituted drug must be stored at 5-6°C to retard deterioration storage makes the solution turbid and to precipitate. There will be progressive loss of activity without increase in toxicity.

Thiopental causes marked depression of respiratory centre and the rate and amplitude of respiration is affected. In small animals it is used for induction or short anesthesia drug is prepared in 1.25%, 2.5%, 5%, and 10% and used depending on the size of the animal. For short duration anesthesia of 10-20 mins dose of 20-30 mg/kg is used. Incremental doses are administered to affect.

In horses injected I/V at 6-15mg/kg after preanesthetic sedation with tranquilizer. Half the dose is administered rapidly and the remainder slowly after the horse is recumbent.

CHLORALOSE

Chloralose may be used for non-survival experiments requiring prolonged anesthesia and minimal surgical interference. There is disagreement about whether chloralose is a true anesthetic agent or a hypnotic with little analgesic action. It is used primarily for physiological studies to preserve the vagal and central baroreceptor reflexes or in acute cardiovascular studies to preserve myocardial function. While chloralose is generally considered to have no application in survival studies or in clinical veterinary medicine one recent study used chloralose repeatedly over a long time period in puppies without any signs of toxicity.

URETHANE (Urethane, EthylCarbamate)

Urethane produces long periods of anesthesia, has a wide safety margin and little effect on normal blood pressure and respiration. It produces sufficient analgesia to allow surgical manipulations. However, the drug should be handled with extreme care as it is considered to be cytotoxic, carcinogenic and immunosuppressive. It also causes profound changes in gastrointestinal function and is stimulatory to the hypothalamus and pituitary.

SAFFAN

Saffan is a combination of two steroids, alphaxalone and alphadolone dissolved in a surfactant (vehicle), Cremaphor EL, to solubilise it. It is administered intravenously or intramuscularly, although the latter route gives more unpredictable results. Muscle relaxation is good and has rapid recovery. It is rapidly metabolized and is an excellent agent for long-term maintenance. It has been used for the cat, pig, large farm animals.

PROPOFOL

Is unrelated to barbiturates, eugenols and steroid anesthetics. It is slightly soluble in water and marketed as aqueous solution. In dogs and cats there is rapid onset and short duration of action and smooth emergence. Is a sedative hypnotic and has minimum analgesic action.

Dose 6-8mg/Kg without premedication in dogs

2-4mg/Kg with sedation

Recovery in dogs is 20 mins and cats is 30 mins

Dose of propofol is decreased by 30-40% after premedication with acepromazine.

The drug is primarily excreted through the kidneys. It is mainly used for caesarian section. Once the ampoule is opened should be used immediately.

DISSOCIATIVE ANESTHESIA

Is produced by a group of drugs which belongs to phencyclidine (it belongs to cyclohexamines), it includes ketamine and tiletamine.

Ketamine

Extensively used in domestic and wild animals, advantage of this is it can be administered I/M also onset is rapid, can be administered I/V also.

Catalepsy is waxy rigidity state and passive state, limbic system is affected it is called as dissociative anesthesia, since the animals are fully conscious occulomotar reflexes, pharyngeal reflexes are present, animal can move its tongue, produces high degree anesthesia. However, muscle relaxation is not there and tonicity of the muscle is present by noticing extensor rigidity of limbs.

In cats 22mg/Kg I/M, 10mg/Kg I/V

Onset of action takes within 5 minutes after administration. The animal loses its righting reflexes and gets to recumbent position, peak affect is reached at 20 minutes after injection and there after recovery starts, duration of anesthesia is enhanced by combining ketamine tranquilizer cum muscle relaxant (ketamine+diazepam= 0.5-1mg/kg I/M) (ketamine+xylazine=1mg.Kg I/M)

On cardiovascular system: Ketamine stimulates the heart rate and Blood Pressure; this is protective for toxemic and geriatric patients.

On respiratory system: At clinical dosage it will not alter the respiratory function. Over dosage may bring about seizures or convulsions. This can be controlled by diazepam or thiopentone sodium.

Use in dogs: 10-15 mg/kg(after premedication)

Since total dose is high it becomes costly. If administered I/V (10mg/Kg) titer the dose to effect. Duration is 15 to 20 minutes, to prolong the duration administer ketamine at 25% of the original dose as I/M. If I/V a little supplementary doses to reach the required plane of anesthesia. Ketamine is not a true general anesthetic but is a good analgesic.

Use in horses: administer xylazine (1.1mg/Kg) and then ketamine at 2.2 mg/Kg, inject I/V, within 10 second after the onset of xylazine action.

Ketamine is indicated for gelding, abscess lancing etc….. Also used as a means of indication of anesthesia and maintenance of anesthesia is by inhalant anesthetic for long duration.

In cattle: Used for anesthesia induction (2mg/kg).

Once the animal goes to recumbancy the anesthesia is maintained by administration of ketamine through I/V drip in dextrose solution.

Tiletamine

Used in wild animal as compared to domestic animals. In domestic animals used in combination with zolazepam (telazole®), duration of anesthesia is 60 minute. This is a long acting drug. Peak effect is seen at 30 mins after injection.

Tiletamine is similar to ketamine, but is longer lasting and more potent; therefore, a smaller dose volume is needed. It is most commonly sold in combination with the tranquillizer zolazepam (Telazol), which improves muscle relaxation, CNS depression, and emergence from anesthesia. It also prevents tiletamine seizures. Cats may take 12-36 hours to be clinically "normal" following tiletamine anesthesia. Tiletamine/zolazepam has proven successful in rats and gerbils, but not in mice or hamsters. Tiletamine causes nephrotoxicity in rabbits.

EMERGENCY SUPPORT

Respiratory emergency

Stop the administration of anesthetic.

Ventilate manually with oxygen at 1-2 breaths/ min.

Resuscitation is important.

Administration of respiratory analeptics.

Maintain patent airway using endotracheal tube.

Cardiac emergency

Administer ionotropic agents like calcium chloride and calcium borogluconate

Adrenaline, sodium bicarbonate, corticosteroids and anti arrhythmic drugs like lidocaine to be administered.

□□□

14

Inhalation Anaesthesia and Agents

General anesthesia was first induced in animals by the inhalation of ether. Almost immediately after the publication of Morton's work on administration of ether to Human beings it was adopted for animals in the Royal Veterinary College, London. Sir. James Simpson introduced chloroform as an anaesthetic in man then it was used in horses all over United Kingdoms.

General considerations of selecting an inhalation agent

- Inhalation agents are vapors or gases administered directly into respiratory system.
- They must absorbed from the alveoli in to blood stream and pass to brain in order to produce a cortical tension (partial pressure) in the brain.
- Inhalation anesthetics are not primarily dependent on body detoxification mechanisms for the duration of clinical effect but or relatively rapidly eliminated by the lungs.
- Because of relative rapidity of uptake and elimination, there is good control of the depth of anesthesia, but constant patient monitoring is required.

Properties of inhalant general anesthetics

1. Nonirritant and free from disagreeable odors
2. Potent: produces pleasant, rapid induction and rapid recovery

3. Produces adequate muscular relaxation and analgesia for surgical procedures.
4. Should not promote capillary bleeding
5. Wide margin of safety – potentially reversible or easily controlled
6. Easily and inexpensively produced
7. Not explosive; stable during storage.

Anesthetic delivery systems

Inhalation anesthetic drugs are pharmacologically active chemicals that cause unconsciousness and changes in organ system function. Their administration requires familiarity with a variety of equipment (vaporizers, flow meters, pressure valves...etc.) needed to vaporize the anesthetic liquid and deliver the anesthetic to the patient.

Methods by which the vapors of volatile liquids and gaseous anesthetic agents are delivered to the animal can be classified in various ways.

Classification

1. Open method (non rebreathing)
   a. Open drop/cone
   b. Insufflation
   c. T piece without reservoir
   d. Induction chamber
2. Semi open method:
   a. Modified ayres T piece (fig.51)
   b. Norman mask elbow
   c. Magill system (fig.52)
3. Semi closed method (Partial rebreathing):
   a. Circle system with pop-off valve open
   b. To - and - fro system
4. Closed method with carbon dioxide absorption

Open (Non-rebreathing)

1. Identification by
   a. No reservoir
   b. No or slit rebreathing of expired gases
   c. Carbon dioxide removal by dilution with room air

Advantages

a. Low cost of equipment
b. Minimal or no rebreathing of expired gases by patient
c. Minimal resistance to breathing.

Disadvantages:

a. Wastes anesthetic: no control of anesthetic being vapourised
b. Difficult to control anesthetic concentration delivered
c. No method to support ventilation
d. Difficult or impossible to scavenge waste gases
e. Vapourisation of anesthetic dependent on room temperature

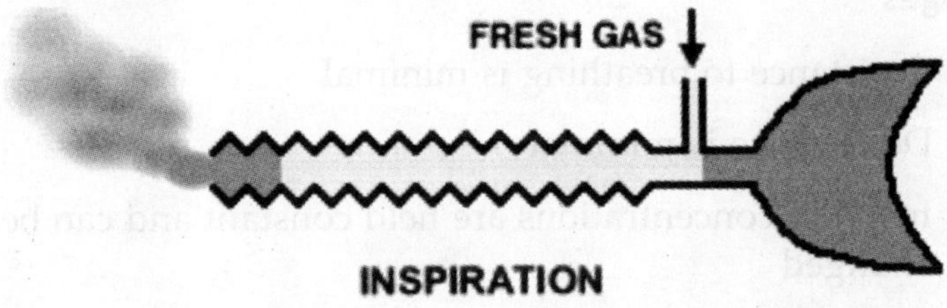

Fig.51. Ayre 'S T-Piece System

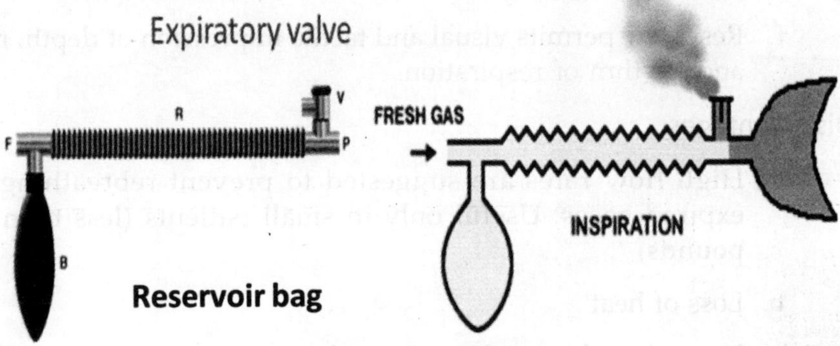

Fig.52. Magill System

4. Precautions
   a. Difficult to maintain stable anesthetic plane
   b. Dilution of anesthetic by room air
5. Semiopen: Here all inspired air is made to pass through the mask on which vaporization of agent occurs.

Disadvantage

1. Difficut to maintain stable anesthetic state.
2. Anesthetic agents are diluted to an unknown extent by air and this dilution is greatest minute volume of breathing is large and inspiratory gas flow rate **is high.**

1. Identification by
   a. Reservoir bag
   b. No or minimal rebreathing of expired gases
   c. Carbon dioxide removal by dilution or non rebreathing valves

Advantages

a. Resistance to breathing is minimal
b. Dead space is minimal
c. Inspired concentrations are held constant and can be rapidly changed
d. Efficient elimination of carbon dioxide
e. Reservoir bag permits assisted or controlled ventilation
f. Reservoir permits visual and tactile impression of depth, rate and rhythm of respiration.

Disadvantages

a. High flow rates are suggested to prevent rebreathing of expired gases. Useful only in small patients (less than 15 pounds)
b. Loss of heat
c. Non rebreathing valve may stick

Precautions

a. Improper valve functioning- check valves for sticky ness and foreign body before use.

b. Excessive inflation of lungs by in flow – watch flow rates and avoid kinking of system.

Semi closed method (Partial rebreathing)

1. Oxygen flow rate depends on patients needs and denitrogenation of the system.
2. Portion of expired gases are eliminated by means of pop-off valve.

Advantages

a. Low gas flow rate is economical

b. Carbon dioxide – absorbent canister is away from patient.

c. Ventilation is readily observed and controlled.

d. Minimal heat loss and drying.

e. Absence of abrupt fluctuations in anesthetic depth.

Disadvantages

a. System is bulky

b. Many parts may be disarranged or may malfunction

c. Resistance to gas flow is greater than with semiopen systems

d. Potential cross infection of patients

Precautions

a. Valve systems can be accidentally by passed or omitted – routinely check machine before use.

b. Channeling of gases in carbon dioxide canister

c. Inhalation of soda lime dust in to – and – fro system avoid use of crumbly soda lime.

Closed system: (fig.53)

1. Circle system with pop off valve closed.
2. Components are similar to semi closed system.
   a. Circle systems with the vaporizer in the circle and vaporizer out of circle.
   b. Higher percentages of each anesthetic may be required for maintenance.

Advantages

a. More economical, Less pollution.
b. Minimal gas flows needed, depending on animal metabolic needs (range: 2-5 ml/lb).
c. Body temperature more easily maintained.

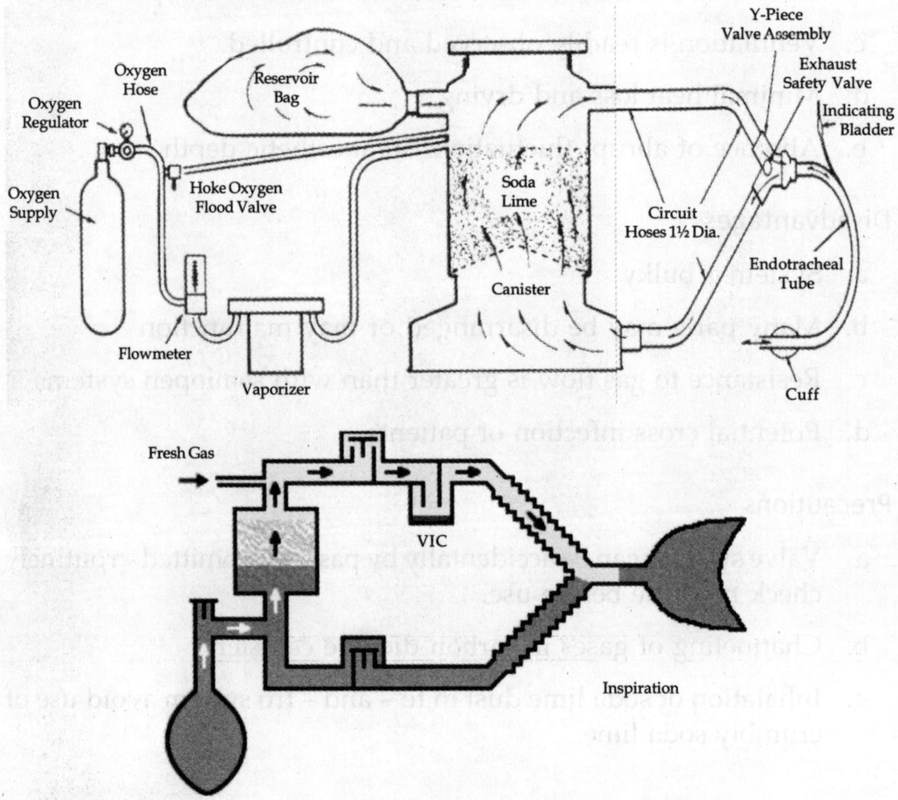

Fig.53. Circle system in Large animal anesthesia machine

Disadvantages

a. Requires close monitoring of anesthetic circuit

b. Difficult to rapidly change anesthetic concentration in circuit

Precautions

a. Virtually no gas escapes from the system: the pop off valve, if present, remains closed – watch pressure monometer for pressure build up.

b. Nitrous oxide should not be used in closed systems unless an oxygen analyzer is incorporated in the system to assure adequate oxygen levels.

Inhalant anesthetic drugs

Classified as

1. Gaseous anesthetics
   a. Nitrous oxide
   b. Cyclopropane
2. Volatile liquid anesthetics
   a) Old generation anesthetics
      1. Chloroform
      2. Diethyl Ether
      3. Ethyl chloride
      4. Trichloroethylene
   b) New generation anesthetics
      1. Halothane
      2. Methoxyflurane
      3. Enflurane
      4. Isoflurane
      5. Desflurane
      6. Sevoflurane

      Volatile Liquid Anesthetics
   c) Old generation anesthetics

CHLOROFORM

It is heavy sweet smelling liquid, which is neither inflammable, nor explosive. boiling point is 61 ‘C vapors are non irritating, easy and not unpleasant to inhale. Liquid is however is irritating to both skin and mucous membrane. It is decomposed by prolonged exposure to light and air therefore should be stored in a cool place and amber colored bottles. Most powerful anesthetic a concentration of 0.035% in blood causes anesthesia.

Effects on:

Heart –dilatation of heart, and decrease in its force of contraction, leads to cardiac failure.

Circulation - peripheral vasodilatation

Liver and kidney - causes cloudy swelling, acute fatty changes in the cells abel to cross placental barrier.

DIETHYL ETHER

It is also called as anesthetic ether. It is a colorless transparent liquid, boiling point 35^0C and vapor pressure about 425mm Hg (20^0C) and highly explosive when it mix with air or oxygen so it is not recommended to use in the vicinity of x-ray room or diathermy units.

It is decomposed by air, light and heat so stored in amber color bottles. It is eliminated through lungs in liver it undergoes bio transformation by forming ethanol and acetic acid. Which do not cause any harmful effect to body. Margin between anesthetic and toxic doses is very wide, so ether is one of safest anesthetic drug.

Systemic drug effects spleenic contraction, intestines become dilate and atonic blood sugar level rises due to metabolisation of liver glycogen because of increased secretion of adrenaline.

Disadvantage

a) It is highly inflammable gas

b) Inhalation provokes secretion of mucous and saliva

c) Post operative nausea is pronounced and animal not eat for several hours after they have been subjected to anesthesia.

ETHYL CHLORIDE

Has boiling point 12.5^{0}C so it is vapor at ordinary room temperature. If compressed it becomes a clear liquid with ethereal smell.

Capable of explosion non irritate to respiratory mucosa used for surface or local analgesia. Fine spray allow to fall on surface, liquid vaporizes and as it does so cools skin about -20^{0}C and fine ice crystals formed over the wound but effect lasts only for 20 seconds.

TRICHLOROETHYLENE

Heavy colorless liquid with a smell which is similar to that of chloroform, having specific gravity 1.46 and boiling point is 87^{0}C so that its volatility at room temperature is low.

It is mixed with waxoline dye,which help to distinguish it from chloroform and less toxic than chloroform.

Preautions

Not use in closed circuits because it release toxic products like phosgene, carbon monoxide… etc.

Advantage: Safe drug, non explosive and non inflammable.

❑❑❑

ETHYL CHLORIDE

Has boiling point 12.5°C so it is vapor at ordinary room temperature. If compressed it becomes a clear liquid with ethereal smell.

Capable of explosion non irritate to respiratory mucosa used for surface or local analgesia. Fine spray allow to fall on surface, liquid vaporizes and as it does so cools skin about -20°C and fine ice crystals formed over the wound but effect lasts only for 20 seconds.

TRICHLOROETHYLENE

Heavy colorless liquid with a smell which is similar to that of chloroform, having specific gravity 1.46 and boiling point is 87°C so that its volatility at room temperature is low.

It is mixed with waxoline dye which help to distinguish it from chloroform and less toxic than chloroform.

Precautions

Not use in closed circuits because it release toxic products like phosgene, carbon monoxide... etc.

Advantage: Safe drug, non explosive and non inflammable.

15

Gaseous Anesthetics

Nitrous Oxide (N_2O)

It is a heavy, colour less gas with a faint, rather pleasant smell. It is non inflammable or explosive but it support the combustion of other agents, even in the absence of free oxygen.

Second gas effect of nitrous oxide

Nitrous oxide has some physical characteristics that distinguish it from other inhalant anesthetics. It has very low blood/ gas solubility, so that its uptake and equilibration throughout the body is very rapid. Because it is used in large volumes (usually more than 50%) and its uptake is rapid during the induction phase of anesthesia, it enhances the uptake of a second anesthetic gas, especially the more soluble inhalant anesthetics, such as isoflurane or halothane.

Advantages

- Non explosive and non toxic can be administered for very long periods with out producing ill effects.
- Provides rapid recovery and post operative complications do not occur.

Disadvantages

- Weak analgesic property when used alone in domestic animal species (MAC is roughly 200% - it is twice as potent in humans).

- Its use together with a primary inhalant anesthetic (such as halothane, isoflurane) only reduces the amount of primary inhalation anesthetic by 25% to 30% of the control value (using halothane or isoflurane alone) at the most. This may not significantly reduce the amount of the primary anesthetic.
- Because nitrous oxide is a weak analgesic agent and must be used in high concentrations, the inspired oxygen concentration is proportionally reduced. This is not suitable for patients with pulmonary diseases that may require as much as 100% inspired oxygen to maintain acceptable blood oxygenation.
- The use of nitrous oxide requires a higher fresh gas flow rate than would be used with oxygen alone. Accordingly the total amount of the primary anesthetic that is vaporized is increased - more anesthetic is wasted, and therefore cost is increased.
- Nitrous oxide diffuses rapidly into closed gas cavities within body, at a faster rate than nitrogen diffuses out of the cavity, resulting in either an increase in volume or pressure. Patients with gastric or intestinal distension (colic, or GDV) or pneumothorax will suffer further. Hence it is avoided.
- Risk of *diffusion (dilutional) hypoxia*. This occurs at the time when the nitrous oxide is turned off and the patient is disconnected from the breathing circuit and starts to breathe room air (21% oxygen). Nitrous oxide is usually used in large volumes during anesthesia (> 50%), and when it is turned off its uptake is reversed and it moves from the blood to the alveoli. Thus, during the first 5 to 10 minutes after discontinuing the nitrous oxide, the volume moving into the lung is large and dilutes the oxygen concentration in the alveoli. If breathing room air, this may result in hypoxia. To avoid dilutional hypoxia, the animal should breathe 100% oxygen for the first 5-10 minutes after discontinuing nitrous oxide use.

Cyclopropane (C_3H_6)

It is a colour less gas with characteristic odor; it is one –and- half times as heavy as air, liquefies at 15^0 C, stored in cylinders made of light alloy without reducing valve. It is inflammable like ether when mix with air or oxygen and is explosive. It causes quick induction and recovery. 8% produces light anesthesia, 15-20% produces good depth of anesthesia.

It shows marked effect on cardio vascular system. It increases hemorrhages at surgical site this is due to vasodilatation. Cardiac arrhythmia can also encountered, this could be minimize by keeping the carbon dioxide content of arterial blood flow at lower levels by effective pulmonary ventilation.

Cyclopropane sensitizes myocardium to adrenaline; it can be safely used in closed circuits danger of explosion could be avoided by mixture of 40% cylopropane with 30% oxygen and 30% helium.

New Generation Anesthetics

Halothane

Halothane is fluorinated hydro carbon. It is a heavy liquid with a specific gravity of 1.86, and the boiling point of 50.2^0 C. It has a characteristic but unpleasant odour. It is not inflammable and not explosive. Decomposes slowly with formation of volatile acids when exposed to light. This is overcome by storage in amber colored bottles and the addition of a small quantity of thymol. Stable in contact with soda lime and thus may be used in closed circuits. 2-4% concentrations vapour used for induction and maintained with concentrations of 0.8-2%.

Absorption, fate and excretion

- Absorption takes place rapidly through lungs.
- Up to 12% of inspired halothane is metabolized by liver microsomes trifluoroacitic acid and bromide and chloride radicals are produced and excreted in urine for many hours to days.
- Metabolites may persist for many days in the liver.
- Major portion excreted via lungs.

Advantages

Halothane is easy to vaporize, and induction and recovery are rapid (1-3 minutes). It is a potent anesthetic, is non-irritant and is neither flammable nor explosive.

Disadvantages

Halothane has a depressant effect on the cardiovascular system. Moderate hypotension is produced at surgical levels of anesthesia because of a reduction in cardiac output and peripheral vasodilation. A dose-dependant depression of respiration also occurs. Some hepatic metabolism of halothane occurs and marked liver microsomal enzyme induction may follow anesthesia.

Special Comments

The desirable effects listed above make halothane an excellent agent for maintaining anesthesia in most species. It should be administered using a calibrated vaporizer since dangerously high concentrations can be attained if a simple apparatus is used. Although recovery is usually rapid, it may be considerably delayed following prolonged, deep anesthesia.

Available as: Fluothane

Sevoflurane (2,2,2-trifluoro-1-[trifluoromethyl]fluoromethyl ether)

Also called **fluoromethyl**, is a sweet-smelling, non-flammable, highly fluorinated methyl isopropyl ether used for induction and maintenance of general anesthesia. Together with desflurane, it is replacing isoflurane and halothane in modern anesthesiology. It is often administered in a mixture of nitrous oxide and oxygen. After desflurane it is the volatile anesthetic with the fastest onset and offset. Though desflurane has the lowest blood/gas coefficient of the currently used volatile anesthetics, sevoflurane is the preferred agent for mask induction due to its lesser irritation to mucous membranes.

In contact with the soda lime in a rebreathing apparatus that serves as carbon dioxide absorber sevoflurane forms at least two degradation products, *Compound A* [fluoromethyl-2,2-difluoro-1-(trifluoromethyl)vinyl ether] and *Compound B* [1,1,1,3,3-pentafluoro-2-(fluoromethoxy)-3-methoxypropane], especially at higher temperatures and when the soda lime is desiccated. Compound A has been shown to cause renal necrosis in rats. In humans, direct histological evidence of renal toxicity has not been demonstrated, although there is dose-related proteinuria, glycosuria and enzymuria. During low-flow anaesthesia, when the lower fresh gas flow leads to decreased flushing of the circuit and increased temperature of the soda lime, Compound A may build up to clinically significant levels. As a result, sevoflurane is sometimes administered with a minimum fresh gas flow of 2 liters per minute, making it a relatively expensive choice for maintaining general anesthesia.

Physical properties		
Boiling point:	58.6 °C	(at 101.325 kPa)
Density:	1.517–1.522 g/cm³	(at 20 °C)
MAC:	2 vol %	
Molecular Weight:	200 u	
Vapor pressure:	157 mmHg (20.9 kPa)	(at 20 °C)
197 mmHg (26.3 kPa)	(at 25 °C)	
317 mmHg (42.3 kPa)	(at 36 °C)	
Blood:Gas Partition Coefficient:	0.6	
Oil:Gas Partition Coefficient:	47	

Routes : Inhalation, via a calibrated vaporiser. Induction dose 5-8%, maintenance 0.5-3%.

Effects

Cardiovascular system: Causes a decrease in myocardial contractility and mean arterial pressure. Has little effect on the heart rate and does not sensitise the myocardium to circulating catecholamines. Does not cause 'coronary steal'

Respiratory system: Causes an increase in respiratory rate; minute volume remains unchanged. Decreased response to hypoxia and hypercapnia. Has a pleasant, non-irritant odour. Relaxes bronchial smooth muscle.

Central nervous system: Principal effect is general anaesthesia; little analgesic effect. Decreases cerebral vascular resistance and cerebral metabolic rate. Increases intracranial pressure in a dose-related manner. Does not cause epileptiform EEG activity.

Toxicity: Trigger agent for malignant hyperthermia

Absorption: Coefficients - blood/gas: 0.6; oil/gas: 47; minimum alveolar concentration: 2.05

Sevoflurane is exceptionally insoluble in blood; alveolar concentration therefore reaches inspired concentration very rapidly, resulting in a rapid induction of anaesthesia

Distribution: Initially to areas of high blood flow (brain, heart, liver and kidney). Later to less well-perfused organs

Metabolism: By hepatic cytochrome P450IIEI to yield hexafluoro-isopropanol, which is further conjugated to its glucoronide. 3% of the absorbed dose is metabolised.

Excretion: Via the lungs, predominantly unchanged. Elimination is rapid due to its low solubility.

Special points: Sevoflurane is unstable in the presence of moist soda lime, producing small amounts of a sevo-olefin called 'Compound A'. Potentiates action of depolarising and non-depolarising muscle relaxants to a greater extent than either halothane or enflurane

Available as: ultane.

Isoflurane

Also called as compound 469 commonly used in human beings. Similar to Enflurane in properties reports till 1975 said it is carcinogenic but later it is disproved boiling point is 48.5°C. molecular weight is 184.49

Desirable effects: Isoflurane produces very rapid induction and recovery from anesthesia and the depth of anesthesia can be altered easily and rapidly. It is non-irritant, non-exploxive and non-flammable.

Undesirable effects: Isoflurane produces slightly more severe respiratory depression than does halothane, but slightly less depression of the cardiovascular system. Its pungent odor has been reported to cause breath-holding during induction in children, but this does not appear to be a significant problem in most species, with the exception of the rabbit.

Special comments: The main advantage of using isoflurane in experimental animals is that it undergoes minimal biotransformation and is almost completely eliminated in exhaled air. This suggests that there will be little effect on liver microsomal enzymes and, hence little interference in drug metabolism or toxicology studies. This characteristic, together with the rapid induction and recovery from anesthesia, has led to the widespread adoption of isoflurane in many research establishments.

Available as: Forane.

Enflurane (Ethrane)

Formula $C_3H_2ClF_5O$

Molecular weight:184.492g/mol

Enflurane (2-chloro-1,1,2,-trifluoroethyl-difluoromethyl ether) is a halogenated ether that was commonly used for inhalational anesthesia during the 1970s and 1980s. Developed by Ross Terrell in 1963, it was first used clinically in 1966.

Enflurane is a structural isomer of isoflurane. It vaporizes readily, but is a liquid at room temperature.

Clinically, enflurane produces a dose-related depression of myocardial contractility with an associated decrease in myocardial oxygen consumption. Between 2% and 5% of the inhaled dose is oxidised in the liver, producing fluoride ions and difluoromethoxy-difluoroacetic acid. This is significantly higher than the metabolism of its structural isomer isoflurane.

Physical properties

Molecular weight	184.5 g/mol	
Boiling point (at 1 atm):	56.5 °C	
MAC:	1.68	
Vapor pressure:	172 mmHg	(at 20°C)
Blood:Gas Partition Coefficient:	1.9	

Methoxyflurane

Methoxyflurane ($C_3H_4Cl_2F_2O$) is an inhalational anaesthetic used in the 1960s, but withdrawn because of detrimental effects on the kidneys. This was due to fluoride ions being produced by its metabolism in the kidney. Its minimum alveolar concentration (MAC) is 0.2, hence it is extremely potent. It has a high lipid solubility (oil:gas coefficient around 950) giving it a very slow onset/offset, thus undesirable for anesthetic purposes.

Synonyms: 1,1-difluoro-2,2-dichloro-1-methoxyethane, DA759, 2,2-dichloro-1,1-difluoroethyl methyl ether, metofane, penthrane, pentran, pentrane, analgizer, anecotan, ingalan, inhala, methoflurane, methoxane, metoxifluran, MOF.

Use: inhalation anesthetic

Molecular formula: $C_3H_4Cl_2F_2O$

Physical data

Appearance: colourles liquid

Mol. weight:164.965 g/mol

Melting point: -35 C

Boiling point: 105 C

Water solubility: negligible

Desflurane

Formula $C_3H_2F_6O$
Mol. weight 168.038 g/mol

Desflurane (2-(difluoromethoxy)-1,1,1,2-tetrafluoro-ethane) is a highly fluorinated methyl ethyl ether used for maintenance of general anaesthesia. Together with sevoflurane, it is gradually replacing isoflurane for human use, except in the third world where its high cost precludes its use. It has the most rapid onset and offset of the volatile anaesthetic drugs used for general anaesthesia due to its low solubility in blood.

The major drawbacks of desflurane are its low potency, its pungency and its high cost. It may cause tachycardia and airway irritability when administered at concentrations greater than 1 MAC.

Though it vaporises very readily, it is a liquid at room temperature. Anaesthetic machines use an unusual anaesthetic vaporiser that heats it to generate a gas.

Desfluorane (Suprane) may increase the heart rate and should not be used in patients with aortic valve stenosis; however it does not usually cause heart arrhythmias. Desflurane may cause coughing and excitation during induction and is therefore used with intravenous anesthetics for induction. Desflurane is rapidly eliminated and awakening is therefore faster than with other inhaled agents.

□□□

16

Anaesthetic Emergencies and Their Management

Onset of general anaesthesia upsets the physiologic equilibrium of the patient and can bring it closer to the threshold of harmful events. If vigilant monitoring is not done anaesthetic procedure can lead to anaesthetic Emergencies and complications. The most frequent time for emergencies to occur is during recovery.

Anaesthetic Emergencies, that require attention includes

1. Respiratory emergencies
2. Cardio vascular emergencies
3. Thermo regulatory emergencies
4. Delayed recovery to full consciousness

1. Respiratory emergencies
   - Apnoea & hypo ventilation
   - hyperpnea
   - Respiratory obstruction
   - Laryngeal and bronchial spasm.
2. Cardiovascular emergencies
   - Bradycardia
   - Hypotension
   - Cardiac arrest
   - **Bradycardia** - As a general rule, for heart rates < 60 beats per min in dogs, and < 25 beats per min in adult horses.

Treatment

- Identify cause and address it
- Dog and cat:

  Atropine – 0.02 ~ 0.04 mg/kg IV

  Glycopyrrolate – 0.005 ~ 0.01 mg/kg IV
- If no response to above treatment, then consider giving isoproterenol 0.5 mcg/kg or epinephrine 0.02 mg/kg IV bolus.

3. Thermoregulatory emergencies
   - Hypothermia
   - Hyperthermia

   Treatment
   - Check airway is patent and intubate if necessary
   - IPPV with 100% oxygen 5-10 sec, ensuring good chest excusions.
   - Assess level of unconsciousness & alter accordingly
   - Analeptic can be used (doxapram 1-2mg/kg i.v can be used)
   - A supply of oxygen
   - Effective carbon dioxide absorbent.
4. Delayed recovery to full consciousness.

Prolonged recovery is occasionally seen in animals with obesity, cardiopulmonary compromise (hypertrophy, shock etc) and some time due to use of glucose during peri-operative period and the effect of preanesthetic.

Laryngeal & bronchial spasm

- Pre anaesthetic Atropine is given i/v as preventive measure
- Oxygen should be administered intrapharyngeally until such time laryngealspasms have relaxed & an endotracheal catheter can be inserted
- Topical application of 4% lidocaine to the larynx.

Respiratory obstruction

- Intraoperatively - disconnect circuit if there is no gas movement, extubate & reintubate with a fresh endotracheal tube. Ventilate with 100 % oxygen
- Pre or postoperatively, if Vomiting or regurgitation is seen then make head downwards and lavage mouth or apply suction to the pharynx.
- If soft tissues are obstructing the larynx, extend the head & neck & pull the tongue forward.

Hypotension

Treatment

- Lighten anesthetic depth
- Fluid therapy
- Provide injectables (e.g., opoids, benzodiazpeines, ketamine, propofol, systemic local anesthetics etc.) to reduce volatile anesthetic requirements.
- Positive inotropes (dopamine, dobutamine, ephedrine) can be administered depending on the condition of the animal.

Cardiac Arrest

Rules of ABCDE

Airway, Breathing, Circulation, Drugs & ECG.

1. **Airway (A)** - Establish a patent (secure) airway as quickly as possible.
2. **Breathing (B)**
   - Attach endotracheal tube to a source of 100% oxygen (preferable to room air, if possible).
   - Administer 6 ~12 breaths/minute.
   - Ratios of one breath per 5 chest compression are used when simultaneously performing chest compression.
3. **Circulation (C)** - Cardiac compression - Place the patient in lateral recumbency on a firm surface and compressing the chest

at a rate of 80 ~ 120 compressions per minute, devoting equal time to compression and relaxation.

4. Drugs used in cardiopulmonary resuscitation

   1. *Vasopressors:* Vasopressor agents given during cardiac arrest aim to improve aortic diastolic pressure. Consequently, increases in coronary and cerebral perfusion pressures enhance both myocardial and cerebral blood flow and improve survival. Vasopressin has been shown to significantly raise coronary perfusion pressures and to increase the return of the rate of spontaneous circulation. It acts on nonadrenergic VI receptors and has been recommended in case of fibrillatory arrest as 40 IU as an i/v single dose.

      Vasopressin acts via specific renal (V-2), and vascular (V- 1) receptors. It produces vasoconstriction in non vital circulations like skin, skeletal muscle, and small bowel, thereby diverting the blood to the brain, heart, and kidneys. The vasopressin analogue desmopressin is mainly a V-2 agonist but has 0.4% of the pressor activity of arginine vasopressin. Plasma half life of vasopressin is 24 min and two thirds of it is metabolized by the kidneys.

   2. *Angiotensine II (AT-II):* Angiotensin II is approximately 40 times more potent than norepinephrine It increases peripheral vascular resistance via direct and indirect vasoconstrictor effects on precapillary arterioles and postcapillary venules. Vasoconstriction is induced by activation of AT-1 receptors on vascular smooth muscle cells. AT-II causes release of endogenous catecholamines from the adrenal medulla leads to peripheral vasoconstriction. Intravenous injection of angiotensin II during CPR further increases already increased serum concentrations of endogenous adrenaline and noradrenaline.

   3. *Endothelin-1:* Endothelin-1 carries potent nonadrenergically mediated vasoconstrictor properties by increasing calcium concentration within vascular smooth muscle cells via a nonadrenergic pathway. It is hemodynamically more advantageous than adrenaline because of lacking beta adrenergic effects. The peripheral effects of endothelin improve coronary perfusion pressure and cerebral blood flow.

4. *Calcium:* Calcium Despite the fact that extracellular calcium enhances the contractile force of cardiac muscle, there is no evidence to indicate that calcium administration during CPR improves cardiac performance. In fact ischemia promotes intracellular calcium accumulation, leading to membrane disruption and uncoupling of oxidative phosphorylation. Because of the risk of calcium accumulation and subsequent cell injury during periods of tissue ischemia, it is indicated when the patient exhibits acute calcium channel blocker toxicity or if there is evidence of ionized hypocalcemia or hyperkalemia. The recommended dose of calcium gluconate is 0.5 ml kg-1 (maximum 20 ml) of a 10% solution of calcium chloride in a dose of 0.2 ml kg-1 (maximum 10 ml).
5. *Amiodarone:* Amiodarone should be considered as a Class lib, following adrenaline, to treat shock refractory VF/VT as early as after three shocks are provided. Amiodarone improves survival to hospital admission but not to hospital discharge because of the side effects such as hypotension and bradycardia.
6. *Procainamide:* It is another alternative to amiodarone but the necessity for relatively slow rate of infusion (30 mg min-1 to a total of 17 mg/kg) makes it a less favorable option.
7. *Magnesium:* The antiarrhythmic action of magnesium is mediated by the activation of membrane sodium-potassium adenosine triphosphatase and blocking of slow calcium channels. Magnesium is universally accepted for the therapy of torsades de pointes. 1-2 g (4-8 mmol) of magnesium sulphate diluted in 100 ml of 5% dextrose is recommended to be given over 30-60 min followed by an infusion of 0.5 -1 g/h. Its use is recommended for shock refractory VF when hypo-magnesemia is suspected e.g patients on potassium losing diuretics, because magnesium mirrors the action of extracellular potassium in stabilizing myocardial cell membrane.
8. *Adrenaline (epinephrine) Adrenergic agonist:* Adrenaline (epinephrine) is routinely used to enhance cerebral and myocardial blood flow by preventing arterial collapse and by augmenting aortic diastolic pressure through alpha 1 and 2 receptors. Its alpha adrenergic receptor stimulating properties

improves coronary perfusion pressure, while its potentially harmful beta adrenergic effects primarily beta 1 actions (inotropic and chronotropic) result increases in myocardial oxygen consumption, in the incidence of ventricular arrythmias, and intrapulmonary shunting due to reduced hypoxic pulmonary vasoconstriction. Accordingly adrenaline increases myocardial lactate concentration and decreases myocardial ATP content. Although beta 2 actions are predominantly bronchodilatory, its stimulation in the myocardium further increases oxygen consumption during CPR and the severity of myocardial ischemic injury after successful CPR.

9. *Noradrenaline (norepinephrine):* Noradrenaline is a potent adrenergic agonist that stimulates alpha 1 and 2 receptors with a minor beta 2 receptor activity, hi contrast to adrenaline it produces greater vasoconstriction such that total peripheral resistance is significantly increased. Increase in both myocardial and cerebral blood flows are comparable with that produced by adrenaline. It also acts on beta 1 receptors and thereby increases myocardial oxygen consumption and the risk of ischemic injury during CPR.

10. *Alpha adrenergic agonist:* Activation of alpha-1 adrenergic receptors result in increased peripheral vascular resistance and myocardial and cerebral perfusion pressure as well as blood flows. Predominant alpha-1 agonists such as phenylephrine and methoxamine, specifically increase peripheral vascular resistance. However, alpha-1 adrenergic is rapidly desentisized in the ischemic myocardium. Stimulation of myocardial alpha-1 receptors increases both inotropic and chronotropic responses leading to increase in myocardial oxygen consumption and this augments global ischemic injury.

11. *Alpha-2 adrenergic agonist:* Stimulation of postsynaptic alpha-2 adrenergic receptors increases endothelial nitric oxide production which counterbalances coronary vasoconstriction induced by alpha-2 adrenergic stimulation. Stimulation of presynaptic alpha-2 adrenergic receptors inhibits the release of endogenous catecholamine, which is beneficial because of the greater levels of endogenous catecholamines during CPR.

There are three subtypes of alpha-2 receptors. Central vasodilator effects are mediated by 2A and 2C, peripheral vasoconstrictor effects are mediated by 2B. It has been reported that a selective alpha-2 adrenergic agonist alpha-methyl norepinephrine without central negative inotropic and chronotropic effects is as effective in restorating spontaneous circulation after untreated VF for CPR and demonstrates less postresuscitation myocardial injury in animal studies.

12. *Atropine:* Atropine enhances automaticity and conduction of both sinoatrial and atriventricular node. It is most effective in hemodynamically significant bradycardia due to vagal stimulation.

13. *Dobutamine:* It is a sympathomimetic amine, which stimulates beta 1 and beta 2 adrenergic receptors and to a lesser extend alpha 1 receptor. It decreases peripheral vascular resistance and increases cardiac output, blood pressure and tissue perfusion. Rapid intravenous administration may cause cardiac dysrhythmias. Dose 0.25 to 20 ug/kg/min in small animals and 0.5 to 2.0 ug/kg/min in large animals (40 to 200 mg in 250 to 500 ml of 5% dextrose or saline).

14. *Isoproternol:* It is a sympathomimetic amine, which stimulates beta 1, beta 2 and adrenergic receptors located in the heart, bronchial smooth muscles, skeletal muscle vasculature and alimentary tract. It decreases peripheral vascular resistance, diastolic blood pressure and mean arterial pressure and increases cardiac output and systolic blood pressure.

15. *Doxapram (Dopram):* It is a nonspecific analeptic agent used to act on the peripheral chemoreceptors. Dose. 0.55 mg/kg I.V. to reverse the effect of xylazine it is administered at the rate of 1.0 mg/kg I. V.

16. *Sodium bicarbonate (NaHCO3):* Bicarbonate therapy should be considered only after the confirmed interventions such as defibrillation, cardiac compression, intubation, ventilation and vasopressor therapy have been ineffective. The bicarbonate therapy should be guided by determining the bicarbonate concentration or calculating the base deficit obtained from arterial blood gas analysis.

    Dose mEq of HCO3=0.3 x base deficit (mEq/L) x Body weight.

17. *Coricosteroids:* These group of agents increases the glucose production, induce hypokalemia by sodium retention. They have inotropic effect on the heart and maintain vasomotor response and suppress the adrenal gland. Indicated in shock and malignant hyperthermia.

18. *Lignocaine:* Indicated in premature ventricular contraction. Only the epinephrine free preparation is used. Dose 0.5 to 2 mg/kg in large animals and 1 to 5 mg/kg in small animals followed by 40 to 60 ug/kg/min I. V. It is contraindicated in slow ventricular rate combined with sinus arrest, sinoatrial block or atrioventricular block.

Electrical defibrillation - Electrical current to convert Ventricular fibrillation into sinus rhythm.

Thermoregulatory emergencies- Hyperthermia & Hypothermia

- Postoperatively the animal should be dried using towels & hair dryers
- Topical heat may be applied using hot –air blankets, infrared lamps or insulated hot water bottles.

If the patient is hypoxic oxygen supplementation is required persistent drug activity can be countered using antagonist drug such as follows :

Agonist	Antagonist
Opioids	Naloxone
Benzodiazepines	Flumazenil
Alpha 2 agonist	Atipamezole

Use of Artificial / Assisted Respiration

These are Special techniques used to ventilate the lungs when the respiratory muscles are paralysed by neuromuscular blocking drugs or rendered inactive by central nervous depression. It is a routine technique in intensive care whenever respiratory failure occurs as in head injury. Commonest method used is **'intermittent positive pressure ventilation** 'of the lungs or **IPPV**.

If the reservoir bag is squeezed as the animal breathes in, the tidal volume may be augmented this is called **Assisted ventilation**.

The increased ventilation produced results in 'washout' of CO_2 and the $PaCO_2$ falls below the threshold for stimulating the respiratory centre so that spontaneous breathing movements cease and the anaesthetist can impose whatever respiratory rhythm is required this is called **controlled respiration**.

Manual Ventilation

When IPPV is carried out by manual squeezing of the reservoir bag this should be done gently and rhythmically. The rate of lung ventilation should be faster than the normal respiratory rate of the animal and the chest wall movement produced should be more obvious than in normal breathing.

Lung Ventilators

These are devices which ventilate the lungs to the required rate, rhythm, pressure & volume.

The changeover from inspiratory to expiratory phase, i.e. the manner in which the ventilator cycles, may be :

a) **Time cycled,** in which inspiration is terminated after a set time.

b) **Volume cycled**, where inspiration is terminated after a preset volume has been delivered.

c) **Pressure cycled**, in which inspiration ceases as soon as a preset pressure is reached.

In cats, dogs, sheep, goats, small calves and small pigs, a ventilator needs to provide tidal volumes up to 1000 ml at a cycling rate from 8 to about 40 cycles/minute. The duration of the inspiratory phase should be about 0.5 to 3.0 sec.

Clinical criteria for ventilators for adult horses, cattle and large pigs are tidal volume of between 2 and 20 litre with a cycling rate of between 4 and 15/min and an inspiratory phase of 2 to 3 s duration.

Complications Associated with Artificial Ventilation

I. Pulmonary

- Ventilator-induced lung injury
- Ventilator-associated pneumonia

- Pneumothorax
- Patient-ventilator asynchrony
- Endotracheal tube occlusion and accidental disconnection
- Oxygen toxicosis
- Tracheal necrosis

II. Extrapulmonary

- Oral ulcers
- Ocular ulcers
- Pressure sores
- Muscle atrophy
- Peripheral edema

□□□

17

Neurolept Analgesic (Opioid + Tranquilizer Combination)

The word neuroleptic originates from the Greek word lepsis ("seizure" or fit"). Antipsychotics (aka neuroleptics or tranquilizers) were investigate by the anesthesiologists De Castro and Mundeleer who coined the term neuroleptanalgesia, an anesthetic process that involves combinig a major neurolepticktranquilizer and the potent opioid analgesic fentanyl to produce a detached, pain free state.

Neurolept analgesia is a condition produced by combination of tranquilizer plus narcotic analgesia which causes sufficient CNS depression to perform surgery without pain.

Most analgesics apart from sedation also produce nausea, vomition, depression etc, to counteract this, neurolept drugs are combined with tranquilizers.

It is neurophysiologically possible to block pain perceptions without completely abolishing wakefulness and without the necessity of resorting to a general inhalation anesthetic. It is this combination of properties that makes Innovar a particularly useful anesthetic agent in the management of certain severely traumatized patients with cranial, brain, and facial injuries and pulmonary complications.

Examples like

1. Immobilon LA- contains etorphine at 2.45mg/ml + acepromazine at 10mg/ml
2. Immobilon SA- etorphine 0.074mg/ml +methotrimeprazine 18 mg/ml

3. Innovar vet- fentanyl citrate 0.4mg/ml+ doperidol 20mg/ml
4. Pethidine and acepromazine can also be used
5. Oxypromazone and acepromazine.

IMMOBILON LA (Etorphine and Acepromazine): is a neuroleptic analgesia which combines etorphine at 2.45mg/ml + acepromazine at 10mg/ml given intravenous in horse. Etorphin is a potent synthetic morphine derivative. Its general properties are similar to morphine. Etorphin is an extremely long acting agent whose effects are maintained by enterohepatic recycling.It provides immobilization and analgesia useful for restraint and minor surgical procedures. Immobilon does not cause excitement, vomition or defecation like morphin. However it acts as respiratory depressant and slows heart rate. Immobilon is reversible in its effects by means of revivon (diprenorphin hydrochloride). Donkeys are more sensitive than horse so half the calculated dose is used in such species.

IMMOBILON SA (Etorphine hydrochloride (M99) and methotrimeprazine): This combination is hereafter referred to as M99 (SA) and consists of 0,074 mg/ml etorphine and 18 mg/ml methotrimeprazine. It can be given by intramuscular or subcutaneous injection. Etorphine is an analgesic which is even more potent than fentanyl (claimed to be up to 1000 times more potent than morphine in some animals). Its effect on the central nervous system varies with species from profound depression to excitation. Respiration is always depressed and bradycardia is common. Onset of effect is rapid and is relatively long acting. Methotrimeprazine, a phenothiazine derivative, is a potent tranquillizer and is said to have analgesic properties. It potentiates M99 and is an antiemetic. Antiparasympathomimetic effects partially counteract the bradycardia.

INNOVAR VET (Fentanyl citrate and Doperidol): used to produce neuroleptanalgesia (it is a state of CNS depression and analgesia prodused without the use of barbiturates and volatile anesthetics). Fentanyl is a synthetic opioid product related to phenylpiperidines. Its analgesic property is 80 times greater than morphin. In dogs, it is used at 1 ml/ 10-15 kg B. wt by intravenous route. This combination is sufficient for minor surgery. The mixture produces sadation, analgesia, immobilization, respiratory depression, panting and bradycardia. Advantage of this drug is easy to administer, wide margin of safety, quick recovery and partial reversibility with opiod antagonists. A mixture of 4-aminopyridine (0.5 mg/kg) and naloxone hcl (0.04 mg/kg) intravenously antagonize the CNS effects of droperidol and fentanyl.

Fentanyl and fluanisone: It can be given by intramuscular or subcutaneous injection, but the latter route is less reliable in all species. Fentanyl is a narcotic analgesic with similar properties to morphine but comparatively high potency (20 to 100 times the analgesic effect). It causes profound depression of the central nervous system, including the respiratory centres in the brain stem, and respiratory depression and bradycardia are produced in most species. Emesis and defaecation, with subsequent loose stools, are common in dogs, and loose stools are usually seen in rabbits and rats for 3-4 days after administration. Fentanyl takes effect rapidly but is relatively short acting. Fluanisone is a major tranquillizer of the butyrophenone group. It potentiates the analgesia provided by fentanyl but counteracts the emetic side effect and partially antagonises the respiratory depression.

Neuroleptanalgesic combinations for dogs and cats

S.No.	Neuroleptic (Tranquilizer)	Neuroleptanalgesic (Narcotic)
1.	Acetylpromazine @ 0.1 mg/kg i/m or maximum total dose 1 mg/ i/v	Oxymorphone @ 0.2 mg/kg i/m or maximum total dose 3 mg/ i/v
2.	Diazepam @ 0.2-0.4 mg/kg i/m or maximum total dose 10 mg/ i/v	Oxymorphone @ 0.2 mg/kg i/m or maximum total dose 3 mg/ i/v
3.	Acetylpromazine @ 0.1 mg/kg i/m or maximum total dose 1 mg/ i/v	Meperidine @ 2-4 mg/kg i/m or i/v
4.	Acetylpromazine @ 0.1 mg/kg i/m or maximum total dose 1 mg/ i/v	Butorphanol @ 0.2-0.4 mg/kg i/m or maximum total dose 20 mg/ i/v
5.	Diazepam @ 0.2-0.4 mg/kg i/m or maximum total dose 10 mg/ i/v	Butorphanol @ 0.2-0.4 mg/kg i/m or maximum total dose 20 mg/ i/v

18

Electro-Anesthesia, Acupuncture Hypothermia & Muscle Relaxants

Electroanesthesia or Electronarcosis

It is one type of analgesia. It is too produced by passing electric current through the brain.

- 1932: Sir Fredrick Hobday- England- He demonstrated electronarcosis in veterinary practice.

  Electronarcosis did not become popular because of some drawbacks

- Sever respiratory depression- leading to respiratory arrest
- During the time of induction there is lot of convulsions
- Margin of safety very less - fatality.

  Indication: short surgical procedures lasting for 15-20 minutes.

Electronarcosis

- Voltage- 40 V AC / DC current
- Current- 35-50 m Amp
- Frequency- 400 cycles/sec

Mechanism

Electrical stimuli activate on opiate/non opiate pain control pathways on brain to produce analgesia. When this pathway stimulated pain tolerant of animal is increases because of this mechanism animals will be under analgesia.

The needle electrodes are applied subcutaneously on either side of the forehead. Then the electric current passed through these electrodes to produce analgesia it is called electronarcosis. The instrument required to deliver AC current is of 40 V, 35- 50 mA and 400 cycles/sec of frequency.

Electronarcosis characterized by

1. Convulsion at the time of induction. To prevent this convulsion use of muscle relaxants before the induction of electronarcosis for smooth induction.
2. Profuse salivation. To prevent salivation atropinization as to done before induction.
3. hypothermia- derailment of hypothalamus
4. Severe stress on the body. It is evidenced by increased corticosteroid levels in blood along with epinephrine level.
5. Decreased blood pressure only for few minutes during induction later it reaches to normal level.
6. Poor muscle relaxation.
7. There will be skin burns, where there is electrodes placed.

Advantages

- It is economical
- Easy to do
- It is performed when other forms of anesthesia or analgesia technique fails
- Immediate recovery after current is switched off.

Acupuncture

It is Latin word Acus means needle

Inserting specifically designed needle at specific points of body for specific therapy/analgesia is called acupuncture.

The specific points where needle is inserted called acupoints/ acupuncture points. This points are shown to be different for different physiological behavior of animals and electrical response of animal and therapy we are going to give.

Acupoints responds to reflex of an organ on the surface of the body and also acupoints are located on imaginary horizontal lines of the body called meridians, which have internal connections with various internal organs. It is reported that there are 14 meridians on surface of the body. Each meridian has more than 360 ocupoints. These points are used for diagnosis, analgesia and therapeutic purpose.

The acupuncture needle is made up of stainless steel, solid shaft and silver coated. Length of the needle will be 0.5"- 5" and 25-34 gauze. Generally for dogs 32 gauze needle is used. In Large animal 21 gauze needle is used.

Hypothermia

Definition

A decrease in body core temperature below its normal value of 37^0 c to 35^0 c or less is defined as hypothermia (mild 35 - 33^0 c; severe < 32^0 c).

Condition where there is decrease in body temperature of animal during major surgeries like brain and cardiovascular system or surgeries of kidney.

In warm blooded animal as temperature goes down the metabolic rate of an cell automatically goes down. There fore the oxygen utilization also reduced. This type of situation needs for surgery of above mention.

How to create hypothermia

1. Surface cooling
2. Body cavity cooling
3. Extra corporeal cooling

Surface cooling

It is achieved by directly immersing animal in ice water or by using cooling bags in which ice water is filled and applied on the animal surface, with this the animal body temperature is decreased. Temperature goes below 20 degree, no anesthesia is required for surgery. Respiration is maintained by artificial ventilation. Blood pH is maintained to alkaline level.

Cavity cooling

It is achieved by pouring cold saline in to the thoracic and abdominal cavity. The body temperature is cooled by repeated pouring and aspiration of cold normal saline.

Extracorporeal cooling system

Running a blood through cannulated artery through the machine.

A hyperthermia system comprising

a) a device for drawing blood from a patient; b) a device for extracorporeal heating of the drawn blood; c) a device for monitoring and controlling the heating of the drawn blood including a temperature probe positioned in the extracorporeal flow of blood, said probe comprising: an inlet end opposed to an outlet end; a flow-directing passage defined by a wall; the wall, the inlet end, and the outlet end configured to define a longitudinal axis; a strut attached to said wall at an attachment site; and a temperature sensor located at the distal tip of said strut to position the sensor in the flow of blood along the longitudinal axis through the passage, wherein the distance from said inlet end to said sensor is less than the distance from said inlet end to said attachment site; and d) a device for returning drawn blood to the patient.

Muscle Relaxants

In large animals centrally acting muscle relaxant glyceryl quaiacolate (Guaifenisin) is combined with barbiturates. 2 to 3 grams of thiopentone is added to 50 grams of glyceryl guaiacolate and 5% solution of glyceryl quaiacolate is prepared using 5% dextrose solution. Anaesthesia can be induced by the intravenous administration of the solution at the rate of 1 to 2 ml/kg in horses.

In dogs succinyl choline, pancuronium, gallamine and other products can be combined with barbiturates. Oxygen administration and intermittent positive pressure ventilation are essential to maintain respiratory and cardiovascular functions.

Procaine and lidocaine

Procaine hydrochloride and lidocaine hydrochloride can be combined with thiopentone and thiamylol. They should not be mixed in the same syringe because the local anaesthetics are acidic and barbiturates are alkaline. Every time the needle or the catheter must be flushed with normal saline before administration of each agent. The advantages are (1) Analgesia (2) Reduce the dose of barbiturates to 50% (3) Protects the myocardium and brain from ischemic changes (4) Act as antidysrhythmic agents and (5) Provide good muscle relaxation.

Long Acting Barbiturate

Pentobarbital sodium is the long acting barbiturate used in anaesthesia and is marketed in vials containing 50 mg/ml and 65 mg/ml. Use of pentobarbital is restricted to small animal and swine anaeshesia. The standard solution is diluted and given intravenously.

Dose

Dogs & cats 20-30 mg/kg without premedication 10-20 mg/kg with premedication. For continuous infusion an initial loading dose of 2-5 mg/kg is given followed by 1-2 mg/kg/hr

A special preparation containing 240 mg/ml of pentobarbital is available and is used for euthanasia of animals. For euthanasia it is administered at the rate of 48 mg/kg (1 ml/5kg). This solution is often used to castrate large boars. The solution is administered deep into both the testicles at a dose not exceeding 24 mg/kg. Castration is performed immediately after reaching light stage of anaesthesia by ligation of the cord and emasculation. The testicles must be disposed carefully otherwise dogs may get access and die due to poisoning.

□□□

19

Post-Operative Pain Management

Postoperative pain is the most undesired consequence of surgery, and if not managed adequately, can lead to delayed recovery. Opioid-sparing techniques are becoming more popular as they decrease the undesired side-effects from narcotic analgesics, especially since data now suggest that some patients who are treated with opioids may have paradoxical reactions, resulting in hyperalgesia, rather than analgesia. Treatment of pain has also moved to the preventive realm, and aims to block the afferent nociceptive bombardment of the central nervous system, before and during surgery. This prevents neurochemical changes that could lead to central sensitisation and chronic pain.

Numerous complications can develop during the post-operative period in small animals. Close monitoring and appropriate management can prevent most of these complications; slight negligence in post operative management will spoil complete process of surgery.

All surgical patients suffer some degree of pain and appropriate analgesia is essential for all post-operative cases. Pre-emptive analgesia (administration of the analgesic prior to the initiation of pain sensation) will provide far better pain control than waiting to initiate analgesia until after the painful stimulus has occurred. The combination of low dose sedative drugs such as diazepam or very low dose acepromazine with analgesics can have a synergistic effect and helps to maintain quiet, comfortable patients.

However, some veterinarians feel that use of analgesics post-operatively makes the animal more active interfering with the healing process. They also feel that absence of pain may lead to self mutilation. This difference in opinion has lead to the non-uniform use of post-operative analgesics in animals.

Pathophysiology: The pathophysiology of postoperative pain is multifactorial, and predominantly of inflammatory nature from skin incision and tissue damage. Inflammatory cytokines, interleukins and prostaglandins produced from the arachidonic acid pathway induce a neuro-inflammatory soup, which sensitises peripheral Aä and C fibres. Ischaemia from retraction of tissue, as well as disrupted blood supplies, contributes to pain significantly, and is characterised by low tissue pH and high lactate levels at the site of incision.

Balanced (multimodal) analgesia: Balanced (multimodal) analgesia uses two or more analgesic agents that act by different mechanisms to achieve a superior analgesic effect without increasing adverse events compared with increased doses of single agents. For example, epidural opioids can be administered in combination with epidural local anaesthetics; intravenous opioids can be administered in combination with NSAIDs, which have a dose sparing effect for systemically administered opioids. Balanced analgesia is therefore the method of choice wherever possible, based on paracetamol and NSAIDs for low intensity pain with opioid analgesics and/or local analgesia techniques being used for moderate and high intensity pain as indicated.

Pharmacological options of pain management

Non-opioid analgesics: NSAIDs including COX-2 inhibitors, Gabapentin, pregabalin

Weak opioids: Codeine, Tramadol, Paracetamol combined with codeine or tramadol

Strong opioids: Morphine, Diamorphine, Pethidine, Piritramide, Oxycodone

Adjuvants: Ketamine, Clonidine

Common analgesic agents used in veterinary practice

- Opioids and Nonsteroidal Anti-Inflammatory Drugs (NSAIDs) may be used for post-operative analgesia in small animals.

Opioids are potent analgesic agents, despite their undesirable side-effects, such as respiratory depression, nausea, vomiting, sedation and pruritus, as well as the possibility of paradoxical hyperalgesia, opioids still remain the treatment of choice for moderate to severe postoperative pain. Their short onset of action, multiple parenteral routes of administration, and lack of ceiling effects (not all of them) makes them very useful in titration doses against pain.

Intraoperatively, nociception under anaesthesia is adequately controllable with potent synthetic opioids, such as sufentanil and remifentanil. It is the conversion to longer-acting and less potent opioids in recovery and the ward which requires a little skill and pharmacological expertise. This often involves administration of a bolus dose intraoperatively, followed by small intravenous titrations in recovery. Although intramuscular administration avoids the firstpass metabolism, and provides a fairly rapid onset, they often result in plasma level peaks and troughs that lead to breakthrough pain between dosing intervals. Increased labour and staffing often contribute to delayed administration of prescribed doses.

Morphine is considered to be the gold standard, single-dose neuraxial opioid. Delayed respiratory depression remains a concern, and these patients need to be monitored in a high-care environment postoperatively. It is also important to note that additional opioids are to be administered cautiously after neuraxial morphine has been given.

Ketamine: Perioperative intravenous ketamine has been used as an adjuvant to treat postoperative pain for decades. Use of ketamine perioperatively makes opioid consumption lower, postoperative nausea and vomition will be decreased and ketamine will be useful in very painful procedures such as thoracic and major orthopedic surgery. The analgesic effect of ketamine will be independent of the type of intra-operative opioid, timing of ketamine administration, and ketamine dose.

Anti-inflammatory drugs: NSAIDs, coxibs and paracetamol are indicated for the relief of mild-to-moderate pain, but given in combination with opioids reduces the opioid consumption, and the adverse effects associated with opioid use. NSAIDs, coxibs and paracetamol are antipyretic, and analgesic, while NSAIDs and coxibs are anti-inflammatory. They work by inhibiting the products of the cyco-oxygenase pathway, both peripherally and centrally. The mechanism of paracetamol is less clearly understood, and seems to work via inhibition of central cyco-oxygenase enzymes, augmenting descending serotonergic pathways, activation of cannabinoid receptors, and inhibiting nitricoxide pathways.

Dexamethasone, given as a single intravenous dose (0.1mg/kg) at the induction of surgery, decreases acute postoperative pain. This is due to its inhibition of the cyclooxygenase and lipogygenase pathways, as well as the inhibition of expression of genes and release of proinflammatory enzymes.

Alpha-2 agonists: Dexmedetomidine, have opioid-sparing, sedative and analgesic properties.

Unfortunately, the analgesic doses of these drugs cause significant side-effects in the form of sedation, hypotension and bradycardia. They are also very long-acting, and can cause delayed awakening after general anaesthesia.

Intramuscular dexmedetomidine (1-1.5 ìg/kg), provides excellent premedication and causes minimal haemodynamic changes. Peak plasma levels are reached 1.5 hours after administration, and analgesia effects persist beyond six hours.

- **NSAIDs** are effective analgesic agents especially in the presence of tissue inflammation. NSAIDs may have some analgesic effect within the central nervous system in addition to the peripheral analgesic and anti-inflammatory actions.
- **NSAIDs** are not recommended for patients that are hypotensive or hypovolemic, have renal disease, gastrointestinal ulceration, diarrhoea or have coagulopathy.
- Drugs like piroxicam and meloxicam, which have higher selectivity for **Cyclooxygenase-2 (COX-2)**, are safer compared to other drugs.

The following are the dosages for some opioids and NSAIDs

Drug	Dosage
Morphine	Dog: 0.2-2.0 mg/kg IM/SC, Cat: 0.1-0.5 mg/kg IM/SC (duration of action 2-6 hrs)
Oxymorphone	Dog: 0.05-0.2 mg/kg IM/SC, Cat: 0.02-0.05 mg/kg IM/SC (duration of action 2-6 hrs)
Pentazocine	Dog: 1-4 mg/kg IM/IV/SC/PO (duration of action 2-4 hrs)
Meloxicam	Dog/Cat: 0.2 mg/kg IM/IV/SC SID
Piroxicam	Dog/Cat: 0.3mg/kg PO SID

□□□

20

General Principles of Chemical Restraint of Wild Zoo Animals

The chemical restraint is generally used to perform painful procedures and examination. Following factors are to be given due consideration before restraining a wild animal.

1. Species, age and sex of the animals
2. Physical condition, status of pregnancy, lactation and status of health.
3. Emotional status and level of excitement.

Any deviation from the normal status in a species has great influence on any chemical restraint procedure. Most drugs are used on body weight basis, and estimation of body weight is an ability to be carefully developed. Smaller species are to be accurately weighed before chemical immobilization.

Methods of Administration

ORAL: Drugs like Ketamine are effective orally, in doses 2-3 times the parenteral dosage. Some caged primates can be made to scream and medicine squirted into the mouth. Though some drug is lost in the process it is still effective. However, the effectiveness of oral medication is often minimal since many of the drugs are either unabsorbed or destroyed-in the digestive tract. Drugs like Diazepam can be used to cool down the animals.

Hand Held Syringe: will be useful especially when the animal is placed in a cage. A luerlock syringe with a large gauze needle is useful in making a quick injection.

Pole Syringe: is a syringe mounted on the end of a pole. It is useful to make an Intra-muscular injection at a safe distance from the animal. Usually the animal has to be in an enclosure and a large bore needle is used to make a quick injection (fig.54).

Blow Guns: are becoming more popular with animal restrainers.

Major advantage of blow gun is

a. Its silent operation with less trauma on impact

b. It can be used in smaller animals

c. Has no mechanical parts requiring maintenance

However it has the drawback of having a short range and the pipe is very lengthy. Blowguns are available commercially. However, a blow gun can be easily prepared using Aluminium, copper, stainless steel or plastic electrical conduit pipes with a smooth surface inside. Usual length of the blow gun is 1 to 2 meters, longer tubes permit greater accuracy (fig.55).

Projectile Syringe or Darts: Modern chemical restraint are made using equipment capable of projecting a syringe to some distance and discharging the contents to the animals upon impact.

The Palmer cap-chur equipment is the standard equipment used in the USA. Other makes from companies like Paxarms of Newzeland, Zooiu Arms from Africa, etc . are also available.

Basically there are three types of projectors (guns)

1. **Short range projector (pistol)**: is a modified pellet gun. It is powered by compressed carbon dioxide. It has a range of around 15 meters. (fig.56)
2. **Long range Projector (Rifle)**: is also powered by compressed CO_2 and has a range of around 35 meters. (fig.57)
3. **Extra long range projectors:** These are powered by percussion caps. The strength of the caps used varies according to the distance from the target. Maximum range is around 80 meters (fig.58). The percussion caps are explosive devices available in four varieties:

a. Very low range **(brown):** has range of 10 to 30 meters

b. Low Range **(green)** : range of 20 to 40 meters

c. Medium Range **(yellow)** : range of 40 to 60 meters.

d. High Range **(red)** : has a range of 60 to 80 meters.

The syringe used in these projectors is specially designed, and is made up of a tail piece, a charge, plunger, barrel and a special needle. When the syringe strikes the target, a small weight in the back of the syringe triggers a charge that drives the plunger forward to discharge the liquid from the syringe.

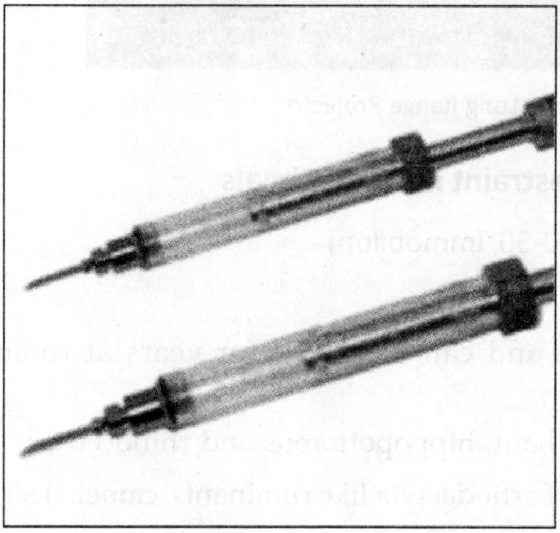

Fig.54. Pole Syringe

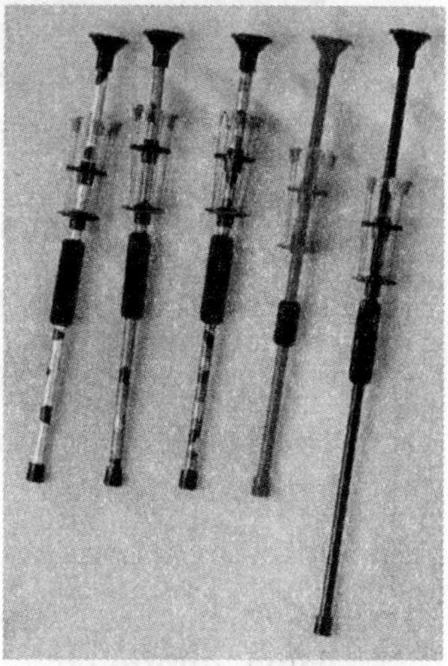

Fig.55. Blow Guns

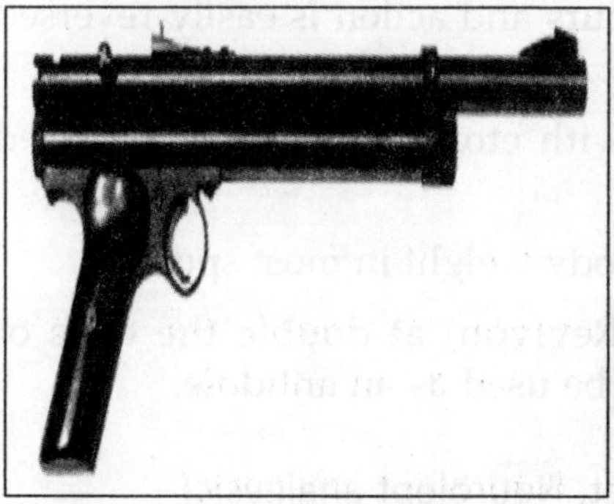

Fig.56. Short Range Projector (pistol)

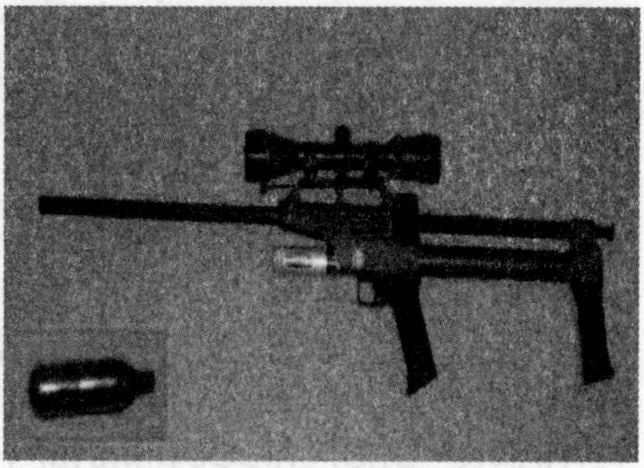

Fig. 57. Long Range Projector (rifle)

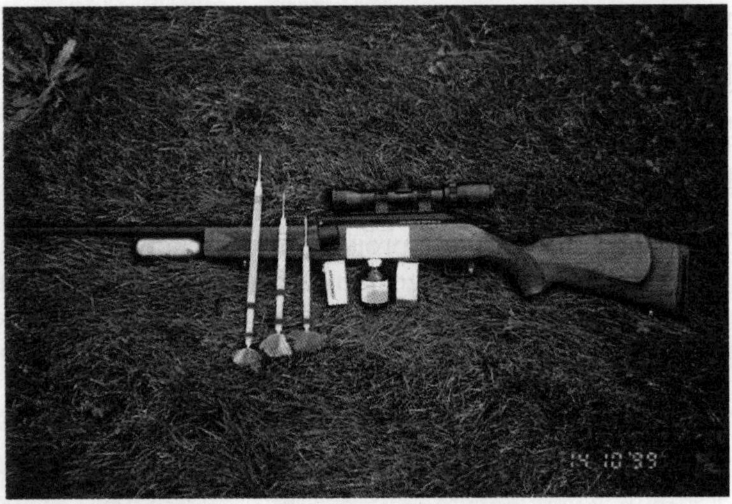

Fig. 58. Extra Long Range Projector

Drugs used for Chemical Restraint in wild animals

Etorphine hydrochloride (M 50-50, Immobilon)

- Is a very potent drug.
- The solution is stable and can be stored for years at room temperature
- Specially useful in elephant, hippopottomus and rhinocerous
- Useful in most species of artiodactyla like ruminants, camel, deer, llama, giraffe etc.,
- Readily absorbed from IM injection, onset within 10 to 20 mins
- Duration of action is upto 3 hours and action is easily reversed with an antidote.
- Atropine is not to be mixed with etorphine (cause decreased solubility)
- Dosage is one mg per 450 kg body weight in most species
- **Antidote** is Diprenorphine (Revivon) at double the dose of Etorphine. Naloxone may also be used as an antidote.

FENTANYL - DROPERIDOL (Innovar vet, Neurolept analgesic)

- Is an analgesic- tranquilizer combination.

- Useful in wide range of Carnivores, Primates and Small mammals
- Useful for short procedures
- In dogs, it is used at 1 ml/ 10-15 kg B. wt by intravenous route.

KETAMINE HYDROCLORIDE (Detalor, Vetalor, Ketaset, Ketmin)

- Is a dissociative anesthetic agent - cause profound analgesia
- Does not produce skeletal muscle relaxation.
- Dosage 2 to 50 mg/kg body weight
- Convulsion is a common side effect, controlled by diazepam (0.5mg/ kg)
- Yohimbine 0.125 mg/kg is antidote.

TILETAMINE-ZOLAEPAM (Telazole)

- Is a dissociative anesthetic tranquilizer combination
- Useful in variety of Carnivores, artiodactyles, birds, reptiles and amphibians
- There is no antidote.

XYLAZINE HYDROCHLORIDE (ROMPUN, XYLAXIN, XYLOCAD)

- Is an sedative, analgesic & muscle relaxant
- Cause depression of CNS.
- Can be used in a wide range of wild animals
- Dosage varies from 0.01 to 2mg/ kg body weight
- Ideal for minor, short duration surgical procedures based on species
- Cause sedation in smaller doses & anesthesia in higher dosages.

DIAZEPAM (CALMPOSE)

- Used to calm down a patient & a good Sedative.
- Useful as an anticonvulsant
- Dosage 0.5 to 1.5 mg/kg body weight.

ACEPROMAZINE MALEATE: (ACEPRIL)

- Is a potent tranquilizing agent, causes depression of CNS
- Causes good muscle relaxation,
- Exhibits antiemetic, hypotensive & hypothermic properties
- Mostly used in combination with etorphine, ketamine & xylazine
- Can be given IV, IM or SC.

OTHER CONSIDERATIONS

- Immobilizing drugs are potent, dangerous and have to be carefully handled.
- Most of the immobilizing drugs are scheduled drugs; legal requirements are to be met.
- Animals that, are recently restrained by chemicals should not be used for human food.

❑❑❑

21

Anesthesia in Laboratory Animals

Rabbit, rat, mouse, golden hamster, Chinese hamster and guinea pig.

Chemical restraint

Numerous drugs used to sedate and anesthetize laboratory animals. The standard technique is to place the animal in closed jar containing a volatile anesthetic agent such as ether or halothane. Anethesia can also be induced with halothane administered via a mask, plastic tube, or anesthetic chamber. Tracheal intubation is difficult because of the restricted space in the oral cavity.

Drug	Rabbit mg/kg	Mouse mg/kg	Guinea pig mg/kg	Rat mg/kg	Hamster mg/kg
Fentanyl-droperidol (Innovar vet)	0.15-0.17	0.8-2	0.08	-	-
Tiletamine-zolazepam (Telazol)	10-25	-	10-30	-	10
Ketamine HCl	20-44	44	20-44	44	-

Intramuscular sedatives and restraint agents are useful in some of the species but not in others. Rabbits are refractory to many restraint agents. Many different drugs and combinations have been used.

The most suitable anaesthetic regime found to be date is as follows

- Acepromazine maleate 16mg/kg I/M. Wait for 5-10 mins then give ketamine hydrochloride 50 mg/kg and Xylazine 3mg/kg I/M. Anaesthesia should last for 30-45 mins. Additional dosage of 50-75 mg of ketamine can be given as required.
- Ketamine used alone will not provide analgesia even with doses of 50 mg/kg.

□□□

DIAGNOSTIC IMAGING

22

Introduction

Deals with production of X rays and its utility in diagnostic and therapeutic purposes.

- Diagnostic usages : Fractures, Obstructions and Dislocations
- Therapeutic : Radiation therapy as in Cancers.

History of Veterinary Radiology, Developments and Advancements

The discovery of X rays was an accidental event during work on Crooks tube in a Physical laboratory. **Wilhelm Conrad Roentgen** (fig. 59) discovered the X rays on November **1895.**

During **1896** first equine foot radiograph was taken.

In **1900** Roentgen Society of United States was formed.

On **10 Dec 2001**,Roentgen received the first **Nobel Prize** in Physics for discovery of X rays.

In **1902** Holz Knecht developed first Dosimeter of Radiation therapy. (fig.60)

In **1913** Gustav Bucky invented grid to remove scattered radiation.

In **1920**- Dr.Hollis Potter invented moving grid. (fig.61)

In **1928** international recommendations on radiation safety precautions were published.

First meeting of The **American Veterinary Radiological society** was held in **1954**; during this period William Carlson was a moving force in developing veterinary radiology in USA.

In **1935**- Substraction technique introduced in radiography by Ziedes de planets

In **1937**- Xeroradiography invented by a physicist Chester F. Carlson. (fig.62)

In 1946- Felix Bloch and Edward Purcell independently discovered the Magnetic resonance phenomena and were later awarded the Nobel Prize in 1952. (fig.63)

In **1955**, the **x-ray image intensifier** was developed and allowed the pick up and display of the x-ray movie using a TV (television) camera and monitor.

By the **1960's**, the fluorescent system was largely replaced by the image intensifier/TV combination.

In **1960 American Board of Veterinary Radiologists** (ABVR) was formed.

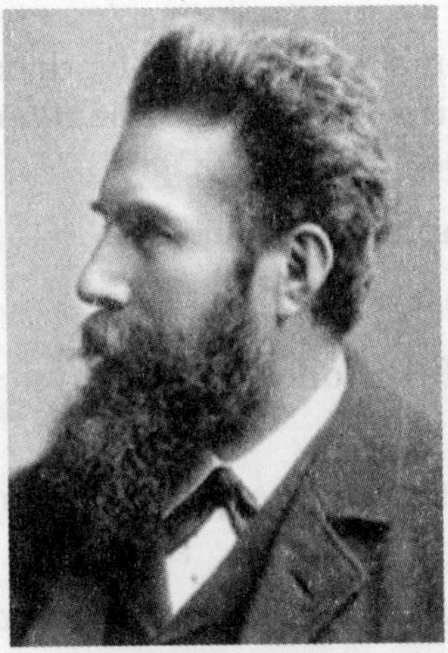

Fig.59. Wilhelm Conrad Roentgen (1895 A.D)

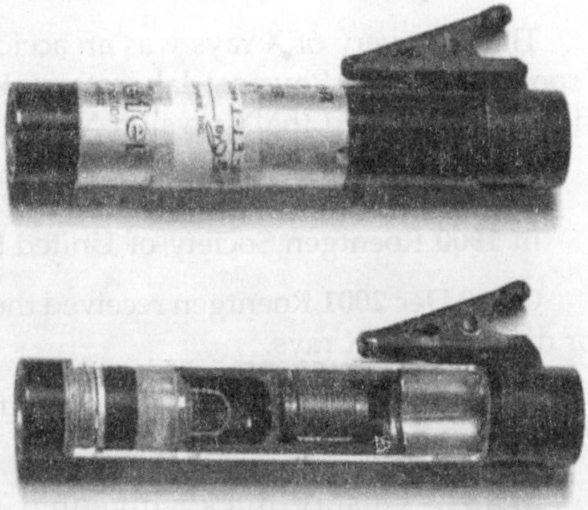

Fig.60. Holz Knecht developed Pocket Dosimeter

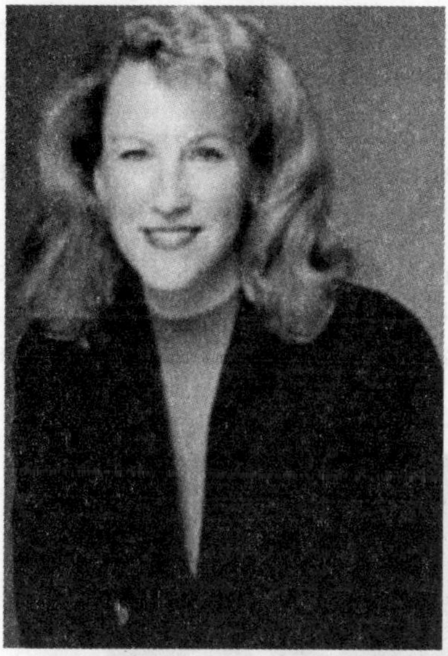

Fig.61. Dr.Hollis Potter invented Moving grid

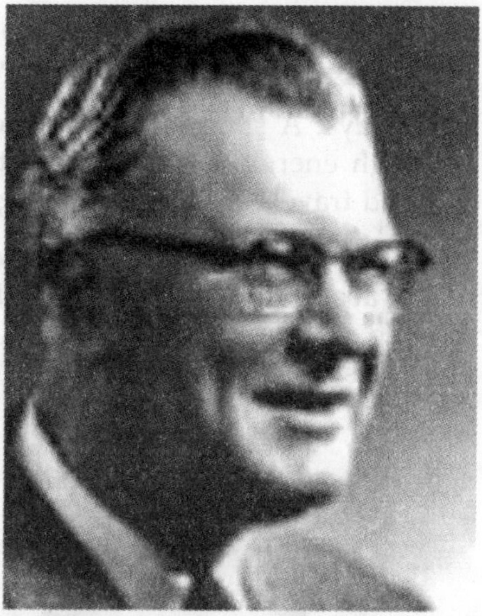

Fig.62. Chester F. Carlson invented Xeroradiography

In **1969** ABVR was renamed as **American College of Veterinary Radiologists** (ACVR).

In **1970- Ultrasound** was invented.

In **1972 - Geofrey Hounsfeld invented** Computer tomography (CT) scan, Known popularly as CAT-scans. Received Nobel Prize in Physiology and Medicine in 1979 for the development of computer assisted tomography. (fig.64)

In **1977- Raymond Damadian** Invention **Magnetic Resonance and Imaging (MRI).** (fig.65)

Definitionb and Uses of Veterinary Radiology

- **Radiology**: It is that branch of medical science, which deals with diagnostic and therapeutic applications of radiant energy.
- **Veterinary Radiology**: It is that branch of science, which uses radiant energy principally for diagnostic and therapeutic purposes in domestic, zoo and laboratory animals.
- **Radiologist**: Any person qualified in medical or veterinary sciences and radiological physics to use radiant energy in the diagnostic, therapeutic and research fields of medicine.

- **Radiographer**: A technically trained person who can obtain quality radiographs for use by a radiologist.
- **X-rays**: A special type of electromagnetic radiation which has high energy, extremely short wave length, no mass or charge and travels at the speed of light.
- **Radiograph**: X-rays interacts with body tissues with some degree of absorption in the exposed tissues. This photographic record of the extent of penetrability of x-rays through the exposed tissue parts is called a radiograph.

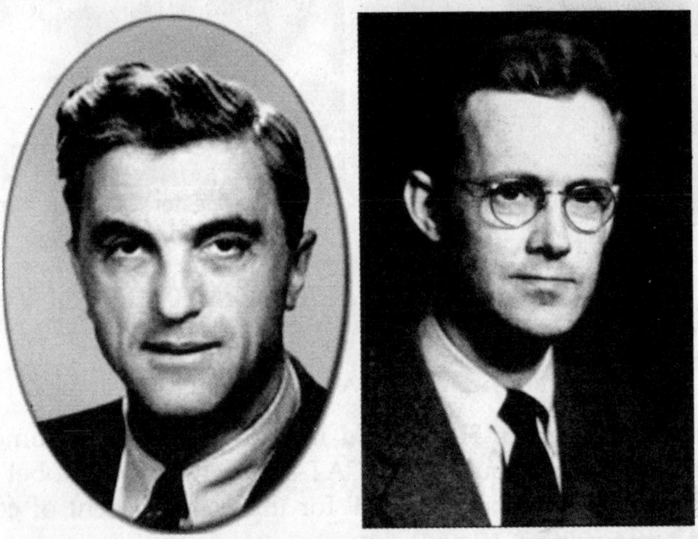

Fig.63. Felix Bloch and Edward Purcell independently discovered the Magnetic resonance phenomena and were later awarded the Nobel Prize in 1952.

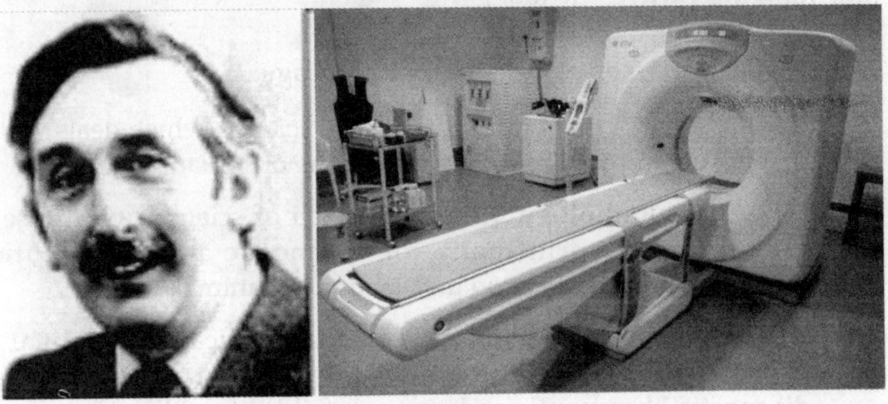

Fig.64. Geofrey Hounsfeld (1972) invented CT scan

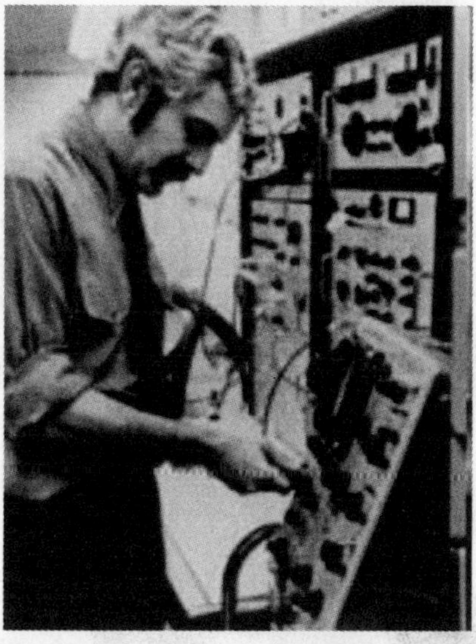

Fig.65. 1977 - Raymond Damadian Invention of the MRI

Uses of Radiography in Veterinary practice

1. As a diagnostic tool eg. Foreign body in stomach
2. To select methods or techniques of treatment eg. for fracture repair.
3. To detect previously unrecognized lesions.eg.Osteomyelitis
4. To monitor the efficacy of a treatment schedule. Eg.,Fracture healing
5. To screen normal animals for morphological evaluation in an attempt to eradicate inherited diseases by selective breeding.eg., Hip dysplasia
6. To determine the age of the animals.eg. Bone growth plates
7. To examine postmortem material.
8. For non-destructive examination of archaeological specimens of animal origin.
9. As teaching aid in the subject of anatomy.eg., Radiographic anatomy
10. In veterinary research eg: osteomedullography to evaluate bone healing.

❑❑❑

23

Production and Properties of X-Rays

Wilhem Conrad Roentgen discovered x-rays while working in his physics laboratory on Crookes-type tubes. Due to the nature and importance of the discovery, rapid progress took place in the production and uses of x-rays in medical science.

X-rays are electromagnetic radiations of high energy and low wavelength produced by the conversion of kinetic energy of electrons into electromagnetic radiations. These rays have sufficient energy to ionize the atom and the ability to penetrate solid matter, animates as well as inanimate, and so are used to examine the internal structures.

X-rays, infrared rays, light waves and microwaves are all examples of group of radiations known as electromagnetic waves. Electromagnetic radiation is a wave motion of electric and magnetic fields. Each EMR has same general form and is associated with extremely tiny amount or bundle or quantum of energy, photon, which depends on the frequency of the wave. Photon is a Greek word, which means smallest amount of energy. The important properties of electromagnetic radiation are:

Wavelength: It measures the quality of radiation and is the distance between the two successive corresponding crests or troughs on a wave :

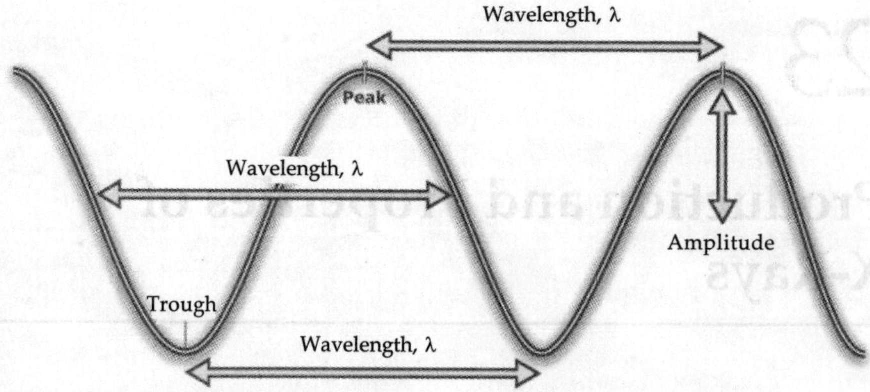

Velocity: It refers to the distance traveled by waves in a second. It is measured in meter per second.

Frequency: It refers to the number of crests or valleys on a wave that passes the point of observer per unit time or identified as oscillations per second or cycles per second. Its unit is hertz (Hz).

Amplitude: It is a function of vigours of wave and is the distance from crest to valley.

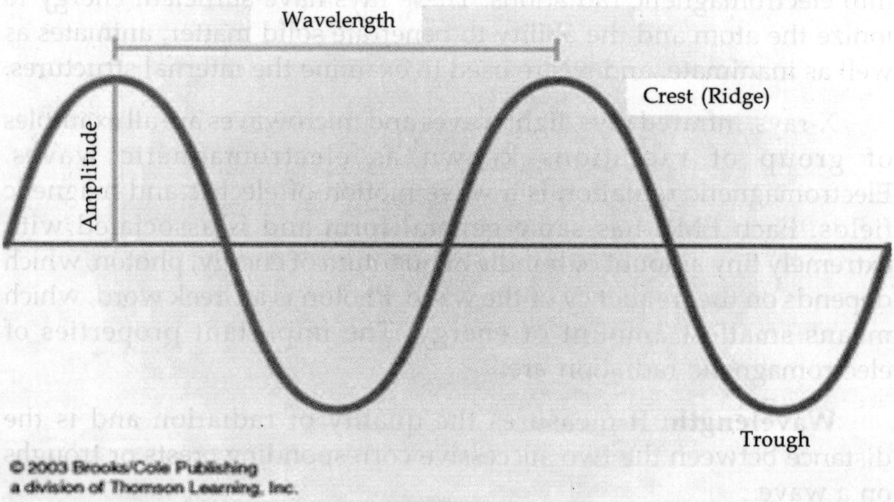

The mathematical interrelationship of these features is:

Velocity = Frequency x Wavelength. In other words, frequency and wavelength are inversely proportional to each other. Higher penetrating x-ray photons have high frequency and shorter wavelength and vice versa.

Properties

- These are electromagnetic radiations and behave as waves. Their short wavelength ranges from 0.1 to 0.5 Armstrong (A^o) with energy levels of 25-125 keV.
- These are high-energy radiations with high frequency. Their energy is inversely related to the wavelength.
- Because of their high energy, x-rays are able to penetrate materials, which readily absorbs and reflect light.
- X-rays travel in straight line with the speed of light (3×10^{10} cm/sec)
- They cannot be focused by a lens
- X-rays do not posses mass or charge and thus are unaffected by electrical or magnetic field.
- X-rays interact with matter, are absorbed or scattered and liberate minute heat on passing through it. Thicker and denser the material more is the absorption and scattering.
- X-rays affect photographic film by chemical reaction initiated in a way similar to that by visible light.
- X-rays produce phosphorescence/fluorescence in certain crystalline materials (eg: calcium tungstate, zinc cadmium sulphide).
- These rays are able to produce indirect ionizing effects on gases because of their ability to remove electrons from atoms. Air is made electrically conductive. The electrical properties of solids and gases are also influenced.

Interaction of X-Ray with Matter

X-ray photon can interact with matter in five ways

- Coherent scattering,
- Photoelectric effect,
- Compton effect,
- Pair production
- Photodisintegration.

Out of these photoelectric effect and Compton Effect are of importance in diagnostic radiology.

Coherent scattering or Classical scattering: Low energy photon (<15KeV) interact with electrons of an atom causing excitation. No reduction in the energy of incident photon and minimum change in the direction of photon. No ionization occurs. It causes radiation fog.

Photoelectric effect: When an incident photon with energy slightly greater than the binding energy of K shell electron encounters this effect. The K shell electron is ejected from the shell. The freed electron flies of as a photoelectron.

- Advantage of photoelectric effect: contrast of the image produced on the film is enhanced.
- Disadvantage is that the photoelectric effect also increases the radiation dose of the patient.

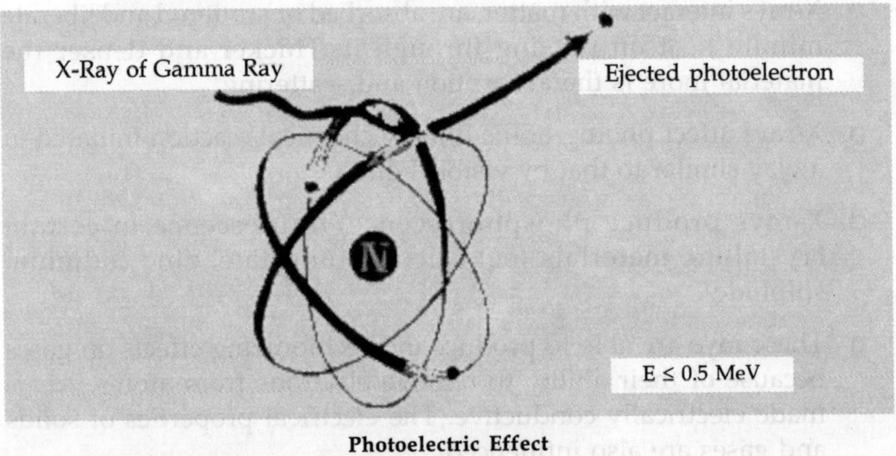

Photoelectric Effect
(Primarily low-energy photon)

Compton Effect: Produced when an incident moderate or high-energy photon encounters a free electron in the outer shell of the atom. Compton Effect produces almost all the scattered radiation in diagnostic radiology.

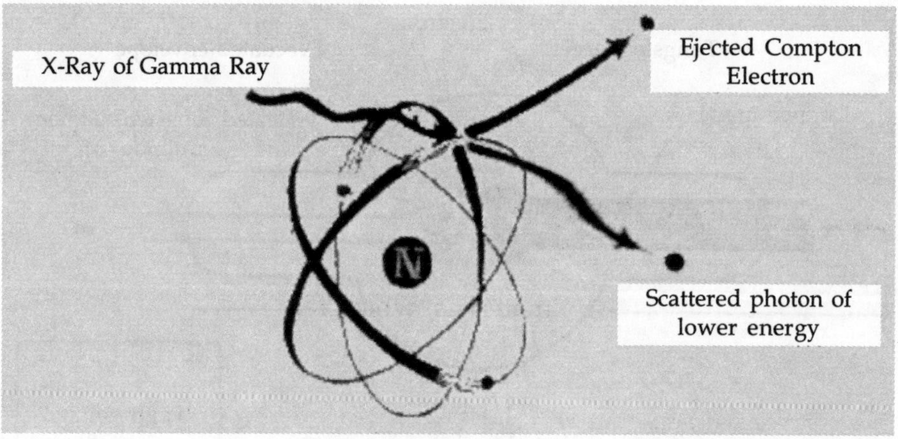

0.5 ≤ E ≤ 5 MeV

Compton Effect
(Primarily medium-energy photon)

Production of X-Rays

If the temperature of a piece of wire is raised high enough, the atoms will vibrate so violently that the electrons nearest the surface will be thrown out of orbits. The process is called **thermionic emission** by heating the filament (2300-2500°C). A very high potential difference is applied across the x-ray tube, so that, the filament or the cathode is given a very high negative charge and the target or anode a very high positive charge. The resulting strong electrical field causes the cloud of electrons near the filament to rush up at high speed through the vacuum tube towards the anode. This stream of electron is called the tube current or cathode rays. The electron stream in the tube is confined and concentrated on a small spot on the anode face called focus or focal spot by a negatively charged **molybdenum-**focusing cup that surrounds the filament. On interaction of these projectile electrons or cathode rays with the target of x-ray tube; operated at the diagnostic kVp range of 40-150 kVp, more than 99% of the kinetic energy of electrons is transformed into thermal energy as a result of collision with outer shell electrons of tungsten (target) resulting in generation of heat in the anode. Approximately less than 1% of the remaining kinetic energy is irradiated as x-rays. Tungsten target has the ability to generate x-ray in diagnostically useful range.

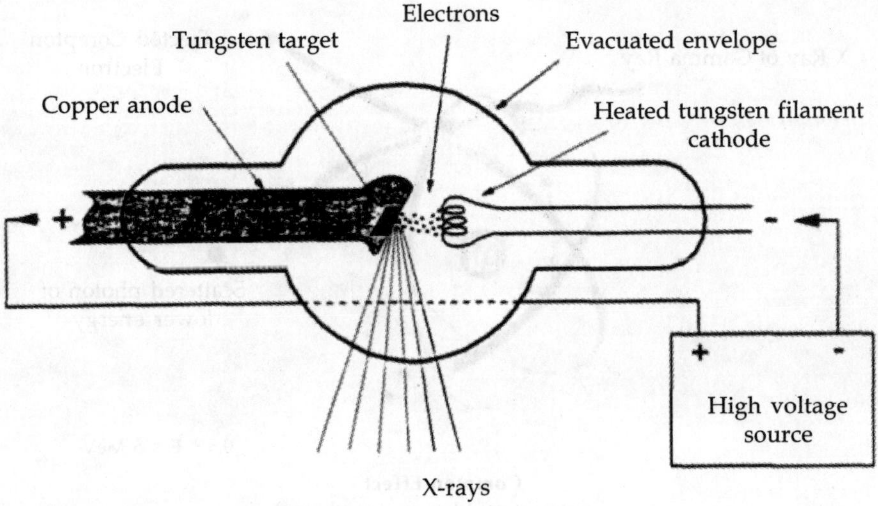

Tube efficiency

It refers to the percentage of kinetic energy of projectile electrons that is converted into x-rays. The efficiency for x-ray production is directly proportional to the atomic number of the target, applied potential difference (kVp) and a large tube current.

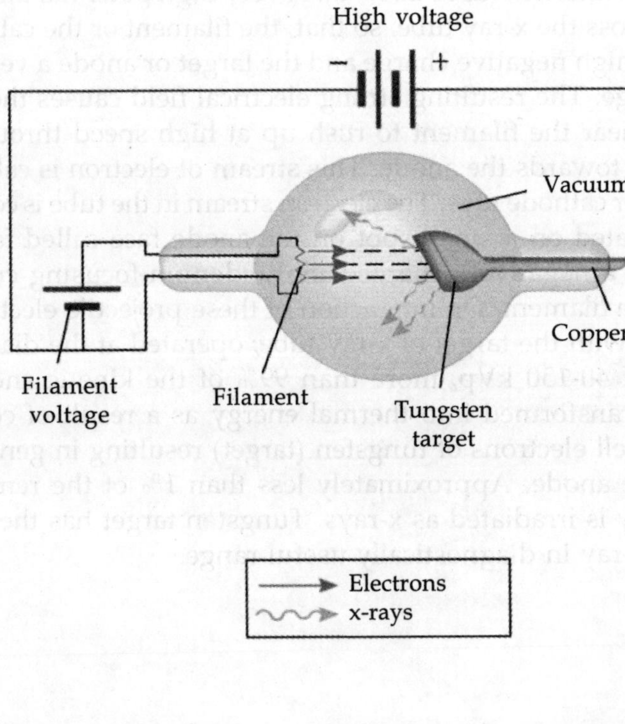

Electron target interaction

An accelerated electron must undergo several interactions with the target atom before losing all its energy. The energy loss occurs through the process of collisional interaction and radiative interaction.

Collision Interaction

It involves the outer electrons of the target and produces heat. An incoming electron may transfer the energy to the target atom or cause ionization. The total energy loss is given off as heat.

Radiative interaction

This interaction is responsible for generation of x-rays. With this type of interaction two types of radiations are given off.

Characteristic or Line radiation

It is produced when the projectile electron interacts with the electron of inner-shell (K-shell) of the target atom. This interaction will result in ejection of electron from the inner shell. When the K-shell electron is ejected, a temporary electron vacancy is produced in the K-shell into which an electron from outer shell or from other atom falls. This shifting of electron is continued until a stable energy state is reached.

X-Ray Machines

X ray machine consists of four parts

X ray Tube – Whole tube is enclosed in a collar of lead except for a small window where X rays emerge out.

- Consists of glass Tube with a high vacuum.
- Two electrode's Cathode (-) and anode(+) are present.

Cathode made up of focusing cup and a filament made up of tungsten. Heated filament which is the source of the electron beam directed towards the anode has High melting point (3370°C), Slow filament evaporation and High atomic number: 74. When exposure button is pressed, an intense electric field is produced between cathode and anode which attract loose electrons away from the filament and propel them at a very low speed. When they collide with the anode they come to a dead stop. Part of this energy is transferred into x rays. (fig.66)

Anode consists of solid bar of copper in alignment with the cathode. Tungsten is targeted to receive the bombardment of electron and it acts as origin of X ray beam hence also called as focus/focal spot. Tungsten (high atomic no. and high melting point (3380°C). Copper serves as conductor of heat from target. (fig.67&68)

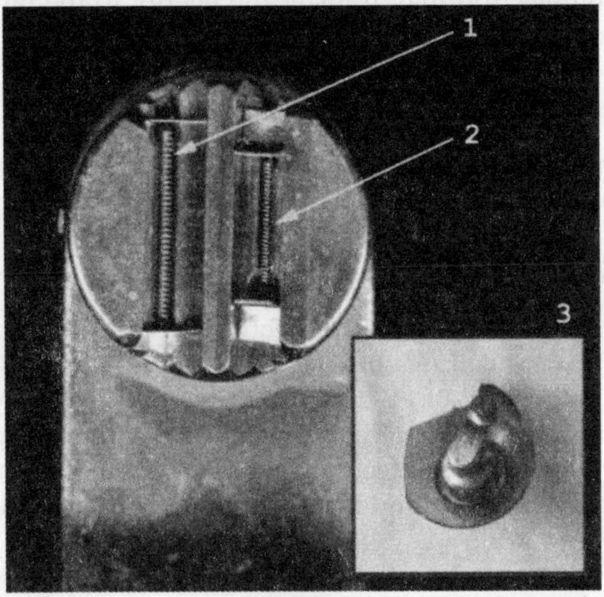

Fig.66. cathode consists of 1. Long tungsten filament 2. Short tungsten filament 3. Real size cathode

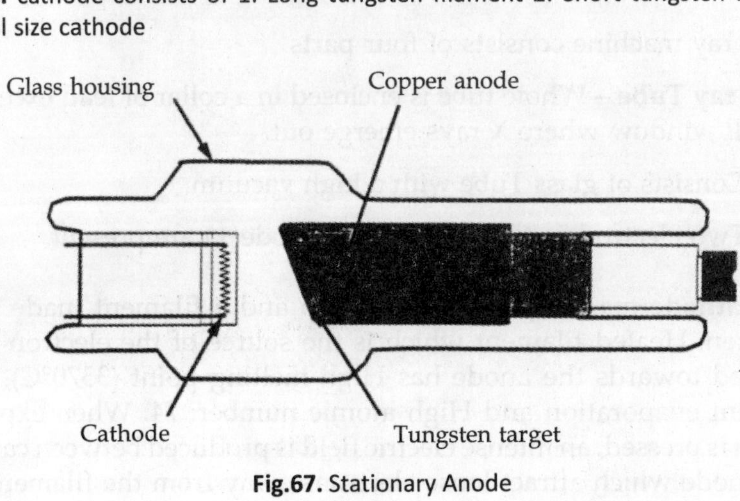

Fig.67. Stationary Anode

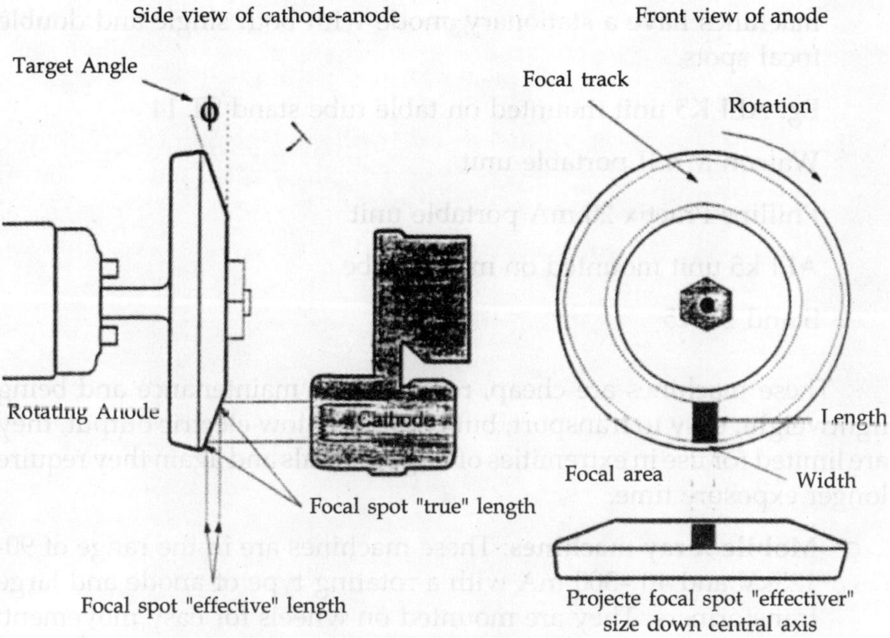

Fig.68. Rotating Anode

Transformers –Essential to convert the current supplied through the mains into a suitable form for the operation in the tube

Tube stand – Form of suspension to support the X ray tube during radiography.

The Control Panel

1. ON/OFF Switch
2. Voltmeter/ Voltage compensator control
3. Kilovoltage selector
4. Miliammeter/Miliamperage selector
5. Timer and Exposure Button
6. Fluroscopy control

X ray machines can be categorized into three types

- **Portable X ray machine**: Commonly used in Veterinary Practice because of their convenience in transportation and handling. It is available in the range of 70-110 kV and 15 to 35 mA. These machines have a stationary anode with both single and double focal spots.

Eg: AEI K5 unit mounted on table tube stand ST 14

Watson MX II portable unit

Phillips Practix 20 mA portable unit

AEI k5 unit mounted on mobile tube

Stand ST 15

These machines are cheap, require little maintenance and being lightweight, easy to transport, but because of low electric output, they are limited for use in extremities of large animals and again they require longer exposure time.

- **Mobile X ray machines**: These machines are in the range of 90-125kV and 40 –300 mA with a rotating type of anode and large transformers. They are mounted on wheels for easy movement.

  Eg: General Electric Mobile 9011

  AEI MR4 Mobile unit

  Watson Mobilix ward unit

- **Fixed X ray apparatus**; These units are in the range of 120- 200 kV and 300- 1000mA.

Special Purpose X Ray Tubes

a) Regular X ray tube

b) **Grid controlled X ray tube:** Cathode, anode and a third electrode called control grid is present which is useful for short repeated X ray exposures eg. Cardiac catheterization

c) **Micro focus X ray tube:** is designed to utilize a Micro focal spot in Magnification Radiology. Micro focus tube utilizes an electron lens to focus the cathode beam to strike a small diameter spot on the anode, produces a fine image detail and eliminates film fogging.

d) **X ray therapy tubes:** operate under low tube current **(5 to 20 mA)** but high kVp settings for a long period of time.

- **Low voltage (50-120 KVp)-** Skin lesions
- **Intermediate voltage (130-150 KVp) –** Lesions few cms below the skin
- **Ortho voltage (160-300 KVp)** – Deep lesions
- **Mega/ Super Voltage (300-1000 Kv)** – Very deep lesions like neoplasia.

Effect of KVP

- Kilo Voltage provides energy for the electrons to move towards the Anode (target).
- High KV strike with a greater impact & X rays of Shorter wavelength (Hard X rays with higher penetrability).
- By altering the KV the wavelength and Penetration ability of X rays could be altered.
- Dense or thick structures requires higher KV.
- Thinner strength requires lesser KV used.

Effect of mA

- mA is the quantity of current supplied to the cathode filament.
- mA should be optimal depending on the area of exposure.
- For larger area and thick parts-more mA is required and for small and thin parts-less mA is required.

Effect of time (Duration of exposure)

- Quality of X rays is also influenced by the duration of exposure (length).
- Generally mili Ampere X time is used as mAS.
- Larger the duration of exposure higher the quantity of x rays.

Collimation

- Restricting the divergence of x ray beam to the minimum
- **X ray Beam:** is an aggregation of X ray photons resulting from millions of collisions of the electrons to the target.

- X ray photon produced at the anode of the X ray tube are emitted in all the directions
- They are confined by the lead shielding surrounding the X ray tube to emerge in the form of a beam.
- X rays with shorter wavelength will be useful in penetration.
- Larger wavelength will be incapable of tissue penetration, but diverge causing the harmful radiations to the patient and handlers.
- This type of x rays should be restricted or controlled by collimation.

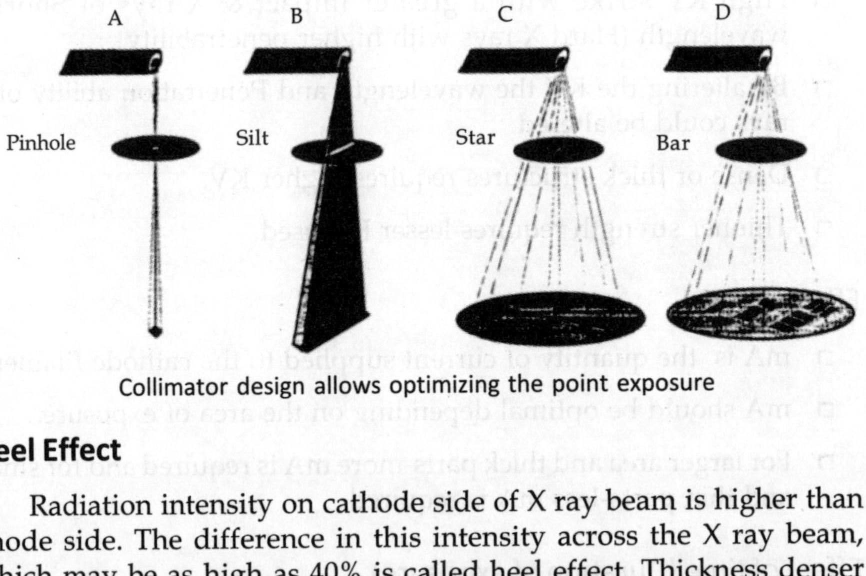

Collimator design allows optimizing the point exposure

Heel Effect

Radiation intensity on cathode side of X ray beam is higher than anode side. The difference in this intensity across the X ray beam, which may be as high as 40% is called heel effect. Thickness denser side should be projected towards cathode and thinner towards anode. Heel effect is more pronounced when large size X ray tube is used and less FFD is maintained.

❑❑❑

24

Factors Influencing Production of X-Ray

The exposed film must be a **'diagnostic radiograph'** i.e.; the area under examination is sufficiently visualized to solve the clinical problem.

Qualities of a diagnostic radiograph

1. Accurate image of the structure under examination without any distortion.
2. Structures must be easily perceptible.
3. There should be no misleading 'artifacts'
4. The four important properties are density, contrast, detail and distortion.

Density

The density of a radiograph is a measure of the light it will let through, when it is held up against an illuminated viewer. It is also called as measure of its blackness. Blackness depends on the number of silver halide that has been turned into silver, which in turn depends on quantity of x-rays.

Contrast

It is defined as the difference between the densities of two adjacent areas (i.e.degree of perceptible difference between two areas) of a film.

- **High contrast**: an image of white bone against a black background with no grey tones.
- **Low contrast** (Flat Film): film with no black/white but only grey.

Contrast depends on choice of exposure factors

1. **Kilovoltage (kV):** affects both contrast and density. If kV is too low, film will have white wash appearance i.e. high contrast and if kV is too high, overexposure and scattered radiation will cause fog. i.e. Low contrast
2. **mAs**: affects film contrast in a negative way i.e. by reducing the contrast when mAs is incorrect. If x-rays are low, film will be pale.
3. **Distance**: Film Focal Distance (FFD) should be 90 cms and Part Focal Distance (PFD) should be near to 0 cm.
4. **X-ray film**: non-screen films have higher contrast than screen films (since intensifying screens increase the image contrast).
5. **Processing**: poor film contrast can result from bad processing (incorrect temperature, time of processing, incorrect replenishment and exhausted developer)
6. **Fog**: shadowing of image by fog can result in low contrast. Some amount of fog is inherent in all emulsions called 'basic fog' and its level should be less than 0.2.

   Fog is caused due to :

   - Over storage of film
   - Premature exposure to x-rays, white light or bad safety light.
   - Excessive developing time or temperature
   - Secondary radiation

Detail

The aim of good radiograph is to represent small structures of the subject with as much clarity as possible. This clarity is known as detail or definition and it will be influenced by the contrast of the radiograph and sharpness of the radiographic image. If objects with definite edged are being radiographed, the film image should have similar definite edge i.e. sharpness. The opposite of sharpness is blur or unsharpness. This may be due to:

1. **Geometric factors**: the size of focal spot, leading to penumbra. The shorter the PFD and longer the FFD, lesser will be the geometric blur.

2. **Photographic factors**: the use of intensifying screens, especially with large crystals and faster ones will cause blur. Second way is by improper fitting of intensifying screen.
3. **Movement factors**: movement of subject has to be kept a minimum. In addition to that movement blur can occur due to movement of head of the machine.

The details of an x-ray image depend for their perceptibility upon their definition or sharpness.

High contrast is required to see very small detail. If one density is merged gradually into another it is difficult to differentiate and if a fine line of demarcation separates it, difference is rarely seen. Blurring of film image affects definition. However certain amount of blurring is intrinsic in any radiograph due to the factors such as size of the focal spot, intensification screen grain size and the lines of stationary grid. The extrinsic factors are movement and magnification; of which movement is the most common cause of lack of definition.

Distortion

To avoid it, part to be radiographed should be placed directly under the center of x-ray beam.

Application of x-rays

Type of X-ray	Approximate energy	Application
Differaction	Less than 10 kVp	Research: structural and molecular analysis
Grenz rays	10-18 kVp	Medicine: dermatology
Superficial	50-100 kVp	Medicine: therapy of superficial tissues
Diagnostic	30-150 kVp	Medicine: imaging anatomical structures and tissues
Orthovoltage	200-300 kVp	Medicine: therapy of deep lying tissues
Super voltage	300-1000 kVp	Medicine: therapy of deep lying tissues
Mega voltage	Greater than 1 MV	Industry: checking integrity of welded metals

The Dark Room

Processing of film in dark room is highly important to get a good radiograph.

Radiographic dark room must be

1. Completely light proof
2. Should not be damp or should not be exposed to extremes of temperature
3. Water and electric outlets must be present.

Light proofing, adequate ventilation (exhaust fans). Walls are painted with white or cream enamel whereas china tiles protect the walls around development tanks.

Dark room equipment

Dry bench

It is the place where cassettes are unloaded or recharged with fresh films. It must be large enough to accommodate the larger cassettes. Top surface is made of either wood/linoleum.

Film boxes are stored in a box. Processing frames are available in different types

- Ilford channel hanger
- Ilford clip hanger

Wet bench

Place where processing of films are carried out. Films are processed in tanks. The capacity of tanks usually is two gallons (9 L). In larger units 5 gallons (22 L) is used. Tanks are manufactured in vulcanite, porcelain and stainless steel, of which stainless steel is the best.

Heaters and thermostats

Standardized processing requires developer solution kept at a temperature of 68ºF (20º C). Temperature could be increased by using tank immersion bath. Even thermostatically controlled water baths are available.

Washing tank

Size should be four times the developer tank with constant supply of water through it.

Drying: Can be dried in a dust free environment or by electric film drier (drying cabinet).

Safe lighting

X-ray film before processing is sensitive to white light. It must be only handled under safe lighting. A safe light is a box containing a low wattage behind a specified filter. Filter is a sheet of dyed gelatin between glasses.

Two types are available

- **Direct:** A diffused light shines directly over the work point (dry/wet bench).
- **Indirect**: The filtered light is directed up to the ceiling where it is reflected over the room.

Safe light is placed in such a way so that work in the dark room can be carried out without fumbling. No "safe lighting" is safe, if a film is exposed to it, too long. It can be tested by holding the film away from safe light at 3 feet distance for a period of 0, 10… 60 seconds and upon development, there should not be any blackening of the film.

Processing of the X-Ray Film

The exposed film is removed from the cassette in safely lighted dark room and placed in a stainless steel plate. It is then immersed in a tank of developer, which completes the reduction of exposed grains of silver halide and makes the image visible. After a specified time, the film is taken out of the developer, rinsed in water and then immersed in fixer bath. This solution removes the unexposed emulsion. The image can now be inspected in white light. After 10 minutes in the fixer bath, the film is washed in running water for half an hour, to remove the processing chemicals and then hung up to dry.

Processing Solutions

For processing standardized solutions are to be used and they should be purchased from a reputable company.

The developer: The exposed film bears an invisible (latent) image of exposed silver ions. The developer solution converts these ions into minute grains of metallic silver

$Ag^+ \rightarrow Ag$

The developing agents first attack and reduce the exposed grains of silver halide, but after that they will begin reduction of the unexposed emulsion causing fog. Therefore developing must be optimum.

X-ray developer

Metol: is a developing agent with high reducing potential. It starts development rapidly and the whole image appears at the same time.

Hydroquinone: has a low reduction potential and is very sensitive to temperature. It commences development on the most heavily exposed areas of the film and produce high contrast.

Phenidine: is new agent, which is replacing metol as the partner of hydroquinone.

Other ingredients include alkali, the preservative to reduce oxidization of the agents, a restrainer to reduce fog, certain additives and water.

Two main types of developers include

- **General purpose**: used for all types of x-ray films. Developing time is 3-5 minutes at 68°F (20° C). Available as powder or as liquid concentrate. Liquid type is more convenient.
- **Rapid working**: used in operation theatre. Developing time is 40 seconds (24° C / 75° F).

Replenishment

Replacing the volume and the activity. A large film will absorb about 60 ml of solution. Developer replenisher is a specially balanced solution made for adding into the developer to keep up the volume and maintain consistent characteristics. Made up solution should not be kept more than three months as they will oxidize and be unfit for use.

Liquid developer

1. **Sodium sulfite**: preservative and also an antioxidant that minimize oxidation of reducer.

2. **Sodium carbonate:** a mild alkali that accelerates the developing process.
3. **Potassium bromide/potassium iodide**: a restrainer to suppress chemical fog and to produce clear radiographs.
4. **Reducing agents** (Kodak Elov developing agent and hydroquinone): to produce metallic silver from exposed silver halide crystals.

The use of cold or exhausted developer solution will lead to under development consequent loss of contrast and definition.

Fixing bath

It contains either sodium or ammonium thio sulphate. When film is immersed in the fixer, unexposed silver halide is dissolved leaving the metallic silver image, which can be viewed, in white light.

Secondly it hardens the gelatin to render it less susceptible to scratches. It also contains an acid buffer to neutralize any developer, which may be carried over.

Clearing time (the time taken for the unexposed halides to be dissolved) depends on a number factors like:

- **Emulsion thickness**: screen films will fix in shorter time than non-screen films
- **Temperature**: warm solution fixes faster than cold. However above 21° C (70° F) staining can occur.
- **Exhaustion**: a load of silver halide in the fixer will retard fixation and hardening.
- **Concentration**: optimum fixer concentration is 40%. Any increase or decrease in this will affect the clearing time.

Chemicals contained in fixer solution include

1. **Sodium thio sulphate (hypo):** it is the clearing agent in powdered fixers or ammonium thio sulphate, which is the clearing agent in liquid fixers. These agents will dissolve and remove undeveloped silver halide from the emulsion.
2. **Sodium sulfite**: it is a preservative and prevents decomposition of the fixer chemicals and helps to clear the films.

3. **Salts of ammonium / alum**: they are hardeners and prevents gelatin fro swelling or softening in the washing water. These salts shorten the drying time.
4. **Acetic acid**: it is usually an acidifier used to assist the chemical action and to neutralize any alkaline developer carried over.

Washing

Washing removes the residual developer and fixer salts from the film which otherwise would attack the image and turns it yellow and faded in few years. A good circulation of water is essential. Usual time of washing is 10 minutes. If the water is hard, a scum can settle on the films, which leads to drying marks. This is being prevented by immersing in a wetting agent (Kodak Photoflo or Ilford wetting agent) before drying.

Other useful processing solutions are

Reducers

When film is either over developed or over exposed and is too dark to interpret and not possible retake the film, the film can often be improved by lowering the density by Farmer's reducer. 20% thiosulphate + 10% potassium ferrocyanide mixture will be yellow. After thorough washing film is immersed in this solution until reduction is brought about.

Source of X-ray exposure

1. **Equipment**: lead shielding, aluminum filter, collimation by cone or diaphragm
2. **Primary beam**: use of collimators, avoid the exposure wearing lead aprons and gloves.

Exposure Factors: Small Animal Radiography

Skeletal system

1. Scapula
   - Posterio-anterior, dorsal with legs extended forward which requires general anaesthesia

- Lateral with the affected side close to the cassette.
- Factors: 5kg – 50kv, 0.3 sec

  20kg – 55kv, 0.4 sec

  40kg – 65, 0.5sec

2. Shoulder joint
   - Posterio-anterior
   - Lateral
   - Anterior-posterior
   - Factors: 50 to 65 kVp, 0.3 to 0.4 sec
3. Humerus: Factors: 45-55 kVp and 0.3 to 0.4 sec
4. Radius and Ulna: -55kv, 0.3 to 0.4 sec
5. Carpus
   - Affections are difficult to detect radiographically. In this case in addition to AP and lateral views, it is better to take medial and lateral oblique views. Use of small cassette and onscreen films are advised to improve the definition
   - Anterior-posterior -strenal
   - Lateral oblique-by adducting the limb
   - Medial oblique-by abducting the limb
   - Lateral
   - Factors: 45-60kv, 0.3 to 0.4 sec
6. Metacarpus
   - Anterior-posterior -animal in standing position keeping the forelimb on the cassette placed at the edge of the tube
   - Lateral
   - Factors: 45-50kv, 0.3 to 0.4 sec
7. Digits
   - Anterior-posterior and Lateral
   - To prevent superimposition, it is necessary to isolate the affected limb.

Hind limb

Pelvis (lumbosacral junction, sacrum and anterior coccygeal)

Hip joint *Ventrodorsal (legs in extension)*

Standard projection for the pelvic area and for evaluation of hip dysplasia. Animal lies on its back, supported by a trough. Animal must be bilaterally symmetrical. Both the hind legs grasped and held caudally.

In case of Hip Dysplasia: use of sedation/General Anesthesia and employment of grid for optimum definition and radiographic methods of identifying the radiographs must be initiated.

Dorsoventral (legs on extension) - Useful in case of trauma where animal resents for extension

Lateral - For reduced dislocated hip. Lateral recumbency with the animal has the affected joint uppermost

Anterior-posterior - Animal lies on its side with femur to be radiographed uppermost extended and held horizontally

1. **Femur:** Lateral: good views of the whole length (Anterior-posterior & Posterio-anterior are also preferred)
2. **Stifle:** Posterio-anterior, , horizontal with animal on lateral recumbency
3. **Tibia and fibula:** Anterior-posterior and Lateral
4. **Tarsus:** AP and lateral
5. **Metatarsus:** Anterior-posterior and lateral.

Skull

Factors: 45-60kv, 0.3-0.5seconds

Canine skull presents problems both in radiography and in interpretation. The difficulty is the variability in the anatomy, which ranges from long nosed dolicocephalic breeds to brachycephalic breeds.

Dorsoventral: more suitable for conscious patients than Ventro-Dorsal (sternal recumbency)

Ventrodorsal: suitable for anaesthetized patients (dorsal recumbency).

Lateral

Nasal chambers: Ventro-Dorsal with jaws open

Temporomandibular joint: Dorso-Ventral view of the skull or lateral view of the skull

Teeth: upper jaw

Dorsoventral -Intraoral

Premolar and molar: oblique view, extra oral

Extra oral open mouth view, lateral projection

Teeth: lower jaw

Incisor area: Ventro-Dorsal, intra oral and lateral, extra oral

Spine: Ventro-Dorsal and lateral

Small Animal Radiography

Soft tissues: Include muscular system and adjacent tissues, pharynx and associated structures, the thoracic cavity, abdominal cavity and the reproductive contents. Because of the slight difference in radio density of various tissues, it is difficult to produce a good contrast radiograph. The use of contrast agents will facilitate the visualization of a particular organ.

Muscular System

Indications

- To show the presence of foreign bodies
- To demonstrate calcification of muscles, tendons or glandular tissues.

Pharynx: Lateral: most informative; 45-60kv

Thorax: To produce a good quality radiograph, following points are to be considered

Elimination of movements (voluntary and involuntary)

a) Use of long FFD

b) Precise positioning

Involuntary movements can be reduced by:

- Use of more powerful type of x-ray machine which takes very little time
- By anaesthetizing and use of relaxants to eliminate voluntary respiration.

Film Focal Distance - 75 cm or 90 cm is used, it will results in considerable enlargement of parts of chest situated away from the film. But increase in Film Focal Distance should be accompanied by an increase in mAs. For chest radiography in dogs 120cm FFD is advisable.

Position: Lateral and Dorso-ventral views.

Abdomen

Problem is identification and demonstration of a particular organ and its differentiation from other abdominal structures. It is because the contents of abdomen are variable in position and often superimposed. Fat acts as natural contrast agent and helps to outline liver and kidneys. Grid is useful in improving the definition.

Movements: can be controlled by use of compression bandage

Position: standing, VD and lateral.

❑❑❑

25

Principles of Viewing and Interpreting X-Ray Films

Radiograph should be viewed in a good, evenly lit viewing box in a semi-darkened room. Image contrast depends upon the intensity of light transmitted through it. Detail may more often be clearly seen by viewing the film from the side than from the front. If the film size is smaller than the viewer, then the bright edges should be masked with black cardboard which improve detail perceptibly.

Provisional diagnosis can be made on the wet film, but to give a final diagnosis film must be dried on a wet film emulsion grains are swollen resulting in refraction of light. When viewing a radiograph, the right side of the film must face the viewer's left side.

Illumination used must be uniform. Otherwise the contrast between areas of viewing box will superimpose on the contrast of the film. Size of the film and viewing box should be same; otherwise viewing box should have adjustable shutters so that only part of the radiograph can be viewed.

In addition to the visual evidence, the data of comprehensive physical and clinical examination of patient should be taken to give a radiological interpretation (sound knowledge of radiographic anatomy set of normal films).

Before Radiological diagnosis the surgeon should be well known with the following details then only the diagnosis should be done: Visual evidence, Anamnesis, Physical examination, Clinical examination, Laboratory results. Radiograph should be multiple views since radiograph is a 2D image of 3D organ. So take at least 2 views 90° to each other. Sound knowledge of Radiographic anatomy with respect to age, Species, Breed etc., is required. Radiograph can describe Size of the organ, Architecture, Density, Position and function. Abdominal and thoracic radiograph are viewed from a distance and bone abnormalities requires Close viewing with magnifying glass if required.

Principles of Interpretation

- Make sure that positioning of patient and preparation are adequate
- Review radiographs in an appropriate environment (lighting especially)
- During lateral view of the body always Head should be towards the left of the viewer
- During VD or DV view, radiograph should be Dorsal or cranial "up".
- Make sure that the radiographic technique is appropriate
- Look for other artifacts (screen blemishes, pressure marks, etc.)
- Evaluate the ENTIRE radiograph, systematically (organ wise)
- Identify radiographic abnormalities (Roentgen Signs)
    - Number
    - Size
    - Opacity
    - Location
    - Margin
    - Shape
- Superimposition - Any shadow that you see can potentially be anywhere in the x-ray beam path. The most common misleading shadows are skin folds.
- Silhouette sign (i.e., border effacement) - Any time two substances of the same opacity come into direct contact, the margin between them is obliterated. Seen most commonly with fluid surrounding soft tissues or two soft tissues which leads to incorrect assessment of size or opacity.

- No metallic objects like collar belts, chain must be present while taking the radiograph.

Radiographic Interpretation

X ray film → Radiograph → Diagnostic radiograph.

Case history

1. Physical examination
2. Correct radiographic procedures
    - Multiple views
    - Positioning
    - Special radiographs
    - Contrast

Radiographic diagnosis

- Location of lesion - Normal anatomical knowledge
- Classification of lesion

Radiographic signs of disease includes

- Size
- Architecture
- Contour
- Density
- Position
- Function

Preconceived ideas may mislead radiographs.

Distance of viewing

Too close viewing of the lesion: abdomen and thorax –may miss the lesions

In case of bones - close viewing and use of magnifying glasses

Use of the spot lights-allows observation of the over exposed areas of radiograph such as soft tissue around bones.

Classification of Lesion

- Developmental
- Metabolic
- Infectious
- Neoplastic
- Degenerative

Types of viewing box

- **Incandescent type**: Pearl lamps arranged in a flat box to form light source with glass or plastic screen. Between the screen and the light source there is glass bottle shield to prevent the radiograph from being heated.
- **Fluorescent type**: has a pair of fluorescent tubes for the light source. Bottle plate is not necessary as little heat is produced.

  Both are available with switching devices to dim the illumination, supports for hanger and tray to catch drops from wet films etc.

Radiographic Errors and Artifacts on the Film

Dark film (high density): Causes of dark film may be Overexposure, decreased film focal distance, increased KVP, increased MA, Long developing time, High temperature of developer or due to Excessive fog.

Weak image or light films (low density): caused due to Under exposure, increased film focal distance, decreased KVP, decreased MA, Short developing time, Low developing temperature, Exhausted developer or due to diluted developer

Fog is an additional density unconnected with primary image which reduces contrast and detail

a) **Generalized fog (film fog):** caused due to use of expired or old film, if films are stored under too high temperature or humidity, if ammonia or other fumes are present in processing room or even by applying excessive pressure on film during storage or handling in dark room.

b) **Chemical fog**: due to overdevelopment of film or may be due to exhausted or contaminated developer.

c) **Radiation fog**: such artifact is seen when the film is exposed to radiation during storage, transportation or during delivery. This makes the image unclear during viewing.

d) Localized fogging at edges.

Distorted images - from improper alignment of the tube, object or film.

Vertical-elongation-vertical angulation too small-foreshortening-vertical angulation too great

Horizontal - overlapping - incorrect horizontal angulation

Finger marks - from improper handling with hands; dark finger marks - developer on fingers - fluoride - particularly stannous - dirt (grease)

Clear finger marks - fixer on fingers

Blurred images - from movement of the patient, film, or tube during exposure. The complete film will be blurred.

Completely clear film

i) Machine not switched on

ii) Malfunction of machine

iii) Placing film in fixer before developer solution

iv) Film not taken/exposed

Cone cutting - beam of radiation did not cover film - improper alignment (vertical or horizontal) or - long axis of rectangular cone placed horizontal for anterior film or vice versa or improper set-up of aligning instruments.

Double exposure - same film is exposed twice. Often this results in another film not being exposed, thus another film will appear clear. The images may appear superimposed, (parallel) at ninety degree angles to each other or upside-down.

Static electricity - films forcibly unwrapped or excessive flexing of film. Seen more often in dry, hot environment. Black "lightning" marks.

Crescent shaped black lines

i) Fingernail pressure on the film

ii) Excessive bending the film

Crescent shaped white lines - cracked intensifying screen.

Reticulation - the emulsion contracts with time when subjected to great changes in temperature between the different processing solutions

Undeveloped / clear area on film is seen due to i) Incomplete immersion of film in developer. ii) Films overlapping during processing. iii) Fixer on operator's hands - clear finger prints iv) Cone cutting sharply delineated round or straight area v) Film not exposed.

Scratched film - Emulsion is soft during processing. Long fingernails, careless handling, during manual processing, wet films touching other films while being processed or drying are the causes.

Black borders – due to Wet or leaking packets allow light to enter a poorly sealed edge of film packet.

Black spots - dirt in the duplicating machine (developer drops will be dark)

Streaks - Improper washing of film hanger.

Radiolucent spots - i) developer drops (dark) ii) powder from the gloves iii) developer chemicals not properly dissolved

Clear spots - i) Air bubbles sticking to film during processing ii) Fixer splashed on film prior to developing iii) Dirt in the intensifying screens.

Brown film: With time the film will go brown if not left in fixer solution or water bath (final wash) for the required amount of time with manual processing. Also with exhausted fixer solution with automatic processing. When the radiograph is initially processed it will appear "normal"

Small, round, irregular, dark dots similar to static electricity - marks due to powder from gloves.

Black film - completely - exposed to light.

Gray film with loss of detail - film fogged - exhausted fixer - insufficient time in fixer solution.

Film image is marred by artifacts caused by dust in the cassette, screen marks, faulty processing etc. If a mark consistently appear on the film, cassette should be isolated, the front of the cassette should be marked 'faulty screens'. Area of poor differentiation may be caused by poor screen contact which could be corrected by judicious positioning.

Abnormal findings in Radiographs

1. Radiograph of GIT tract of cat with Barium showing roundworm (fig. 69).
2. Radiograph shows intestinal foreign body and on exploration it was found that the foreign body was corn cob. (fig. 70)
3. Radiograph showing Intestinal obstruction caused by marble stone. (fig. 71)
4. Radiograph showing gastro-pyloro-dueodenal obstruction caused by linear foreign body in a pregnant dog. (fig. 72)
5. Radiograph showing intestinal obstruction caused by jackfruit seed. (fig. 73)
6. Radiograph Showing Intussusception in a dog. (fig. 74)
7. Radiograph showing foreign body in thoracic cavity. (fig. 75)
8. Radiograph showing bone pieces in the stomach and intestine. (fig. 76)
9. Radiograph showing solitary cystolith in bladder. (fig. 77)

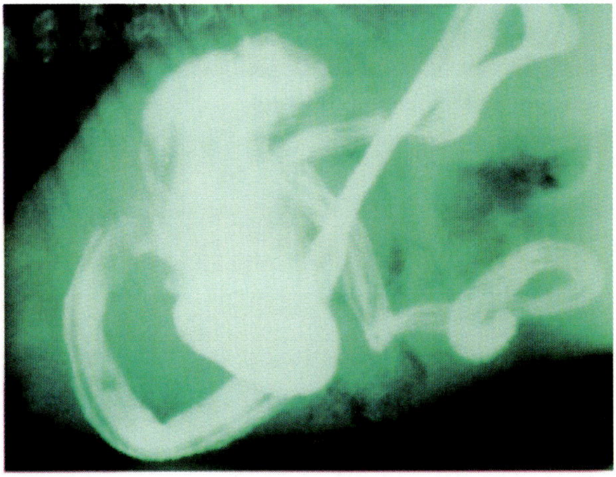

Fig.69. Radiograph of GIT tract of cat with Barium showing roundworm

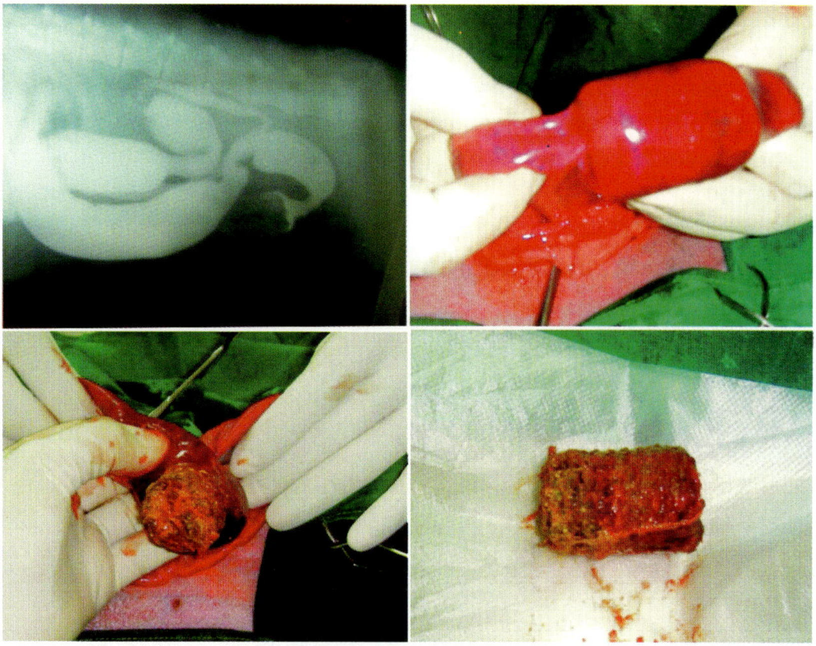

Fig.70. Radiograph shows intestinal foreign body (corn cob)

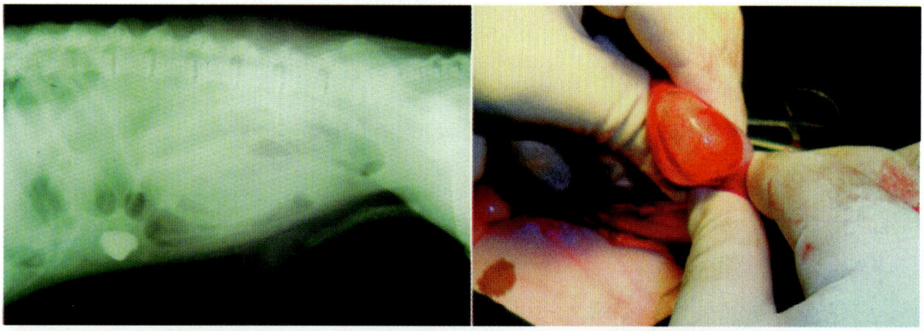

Fig.71. Radiograph showing Intestinal obstruction caused by marble stone in dog

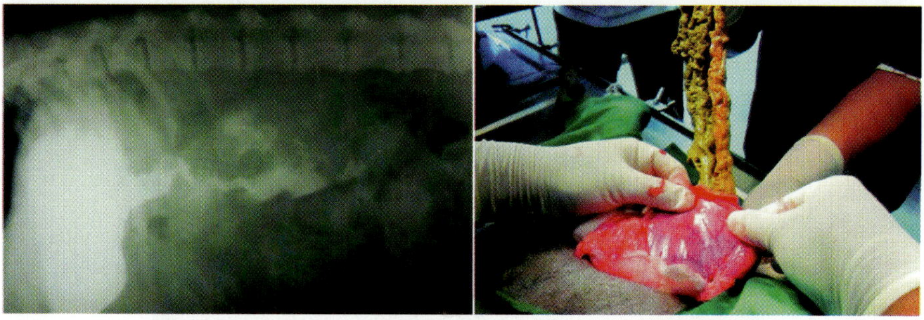

Fig.72. Radiograph showing gastro-pyloro-dueodenal obstruction caused by linear foreign body in a pregnant dog

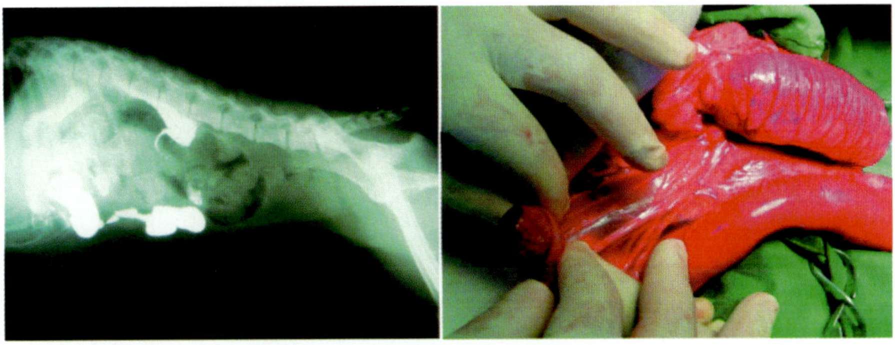

Fig.73. Radiograph showing intestinal obstruction caused by jackfruit seed

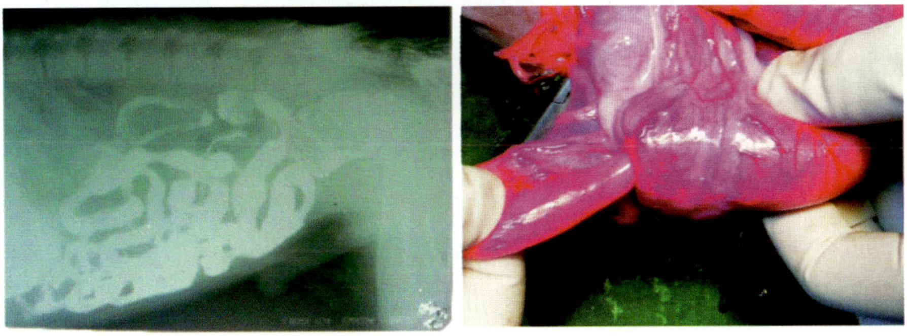

Fig.74. Radiograph showing Intussusception in a dog

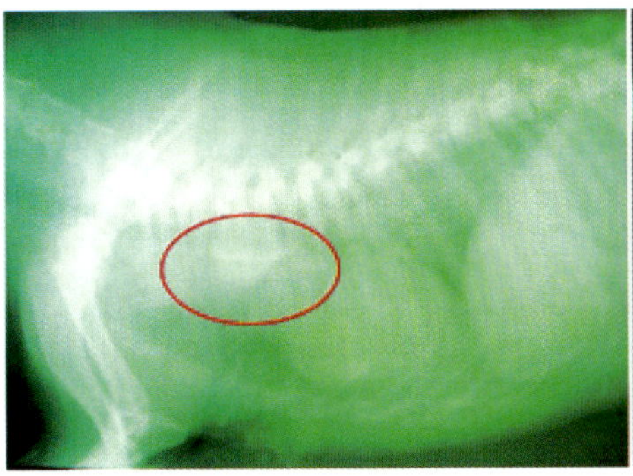

Fig.75. Radiograph showing foreign body in thoracic cavity

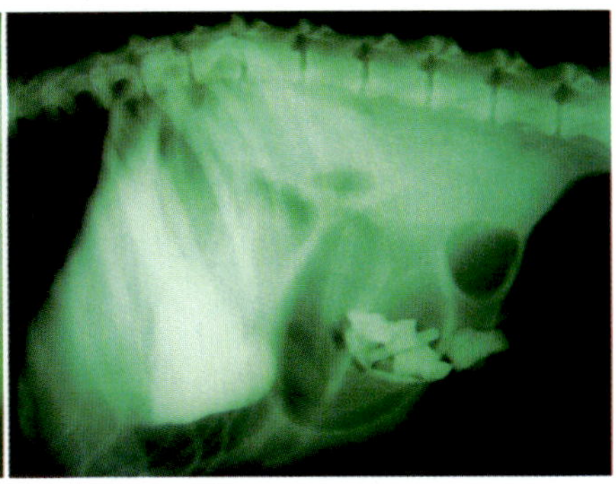

Fig.76. Radiograph showing bone pieces in the stomach and intestine

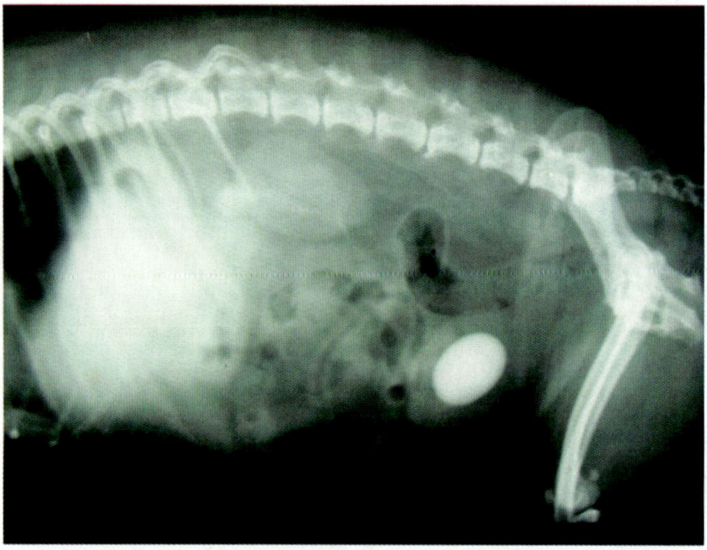

Fig.77. Radiograph showing solitary cystolith in bladder

❑❑❑

26

Contrast Radiography

During the radiography of soft tissues, it is often difficult to visualize a particular organ owing to its lack of contrast with the surrounding tissues. In these circumstances, the use of contrast medium is helpful to outline the structure.

The substances employed for this purpose are usually of high atomic number (compounds of barium and iodine). Since such substance is relatively radio opaque to x-rays. Occasionally gases of low density and more transparent to x-rays are employed. These substances are either administered to fill the organ or made to excrete through the organ to be demonstrated. These agents are classified into 5 main groups

1. **Agents employed for the demonstration of alimentary tract:** substance used must be completely insoluble with no possibility of they being absorbed through the bowel wall. Eg: barium sulphate – prepared in a fine colloidal form, which provide optimum outlining of the mucosal pattern. Main disadvantage is that if they are introduced into the trachea or pass to peritoneum they will not be absorbed or eliminated and they remain in situ indefinitely
2. **Water-soluble agents**: they are organic iodine preparations since they are water soluble, gets rapidly eliminated after introduction into the body. They are injected into vascular system, either for immediate visualization of the system or for subsequent demonstration of urinary system during their excretion through kidneys. These agents in human's causes side effects in number

of patients like flushing of the face, palpitations, slight unconsciousness and nausea. In sever cases, abdominal pain, vomition, instances of development of shock and death are also reported. Hence test dose is administered before actual use. The side effects are either due to allergy to preparation or drug idiosyncrasy. These agents are administered directly into the vascular system as in any tissue it may cause irritation.

3. **Agents excreted into the biliary system (Cholecystopaque):** usually organic iodine preparations which after absorption from the alimentary tract or following i/v injection are largely excreted by the liver and visualize biliary system

4. **Viscous and oily agents**: viscous forms are used for slow excretion especially in bronchial tree and uterus. Oily preparation are used to void even the slightest chance of irritation and once administered they are slowly eliminated.

5. **Gaseous agents**: among the gases, air and oxygen are frequently employed. They are cheap, easy to administer and comparatively safe.

The tissue itself or its surrounding structure is deliberately altered to obtain a radiograph with enhanced visualization and demarcation. It is called contrast radiography and the substances needed for this purpose is called contrast medium.

Positive contrast: materials, which increase the radio density of structure or tissue in relation to surrounding tissue.

Negative contrast: materials, which decrease radio density of structure or tissue in relation to surrounding tissue..

Double contrast: use of both positive and negative contrast.

By contrast radiography, size, shape, position, serosal and mucosal pattern of hollow organs and functions of organs can be studied more significantly.

Positive contrast media

Atomic number (Z)-radio density Z of bone-138, Air- 40

For contrast agent Z should be >50 barium-56, Iodine-53

Contrast medium

- Desired atomic number
- Inert and non toxic: lead (Z=82) lead oxide in soap water in experimental animals)
- Excretory type-retention in organs for a reliable time

Adverse effects

- **Chemo toxic/localized**: urticarea, muscle jerks etc
- **Systemic /hypersensitive**: coma in renal/cardiac abnormalities, diabetes mellitus and dehydration

Negative contrast media

Commonly air and CO_2 are used

Nitrogen is a negative contrast media which is inert, quickly dissolve in body fluids and rapidly eliminated from the body

Used for arthrography, fasciography, pneumoperitonium, pneumocystography etc

Water-soluble preparations

Generic name	Trade name	Iodine Mg/ml	I/NI	Uses
Meglumine iothalamate	Conray 280	280	I	
Sodium iothalamate	Conray 420	420	I	Angiography, osteomedullography, sialography, Intravenous pyelography, uretreogarphy, arthrogarphy
Meglumine diatrizoate	Hyapque 65%	390	I	
Sodium diatrizoate	Urograffin290	290	I	
	Urograffin 370	370	I	
	Renograffin 60	60	I	
	Renograffin 70	70	I	
Metrizamide	Amipaque	300	NI	
Iopamidol	Niopam 200	200	NI	
	Niopam 300	300	NI	Myelography, IVP, arthrography
	Niopam 370	370	NI	
Iohexol	Omnipaque 140	140	NI	
	Omnipaque 180	180	NI	

	Omnipaque 300	300	NI	
	Omnipaque 350	350	NI	
Viscous and oily preparation				
	Dianosil aqueous	280		Lymphangiography,
Propylidione	Dianosil oily	340		dacrocystorhinnography,
Iodized poppy seed oil	Lipiodol-ultra	480		hysterosalphingography Myelography
Iophendylate	Myodil	300		Bronchography Sialography
Barium sulphate preparations				
Barium sulphate suspension	Micropaque Standard Baritop 100 Microbar suspension			
Barium sulphate powder	Micropaque HD(High-Density) Baritop G Microtrast			Esophagus, gastrography, reticulography, barium meals, barium enema
Barium sulphate paste	Microtrast			
Preparation excreted through biliary system				
Iopanoic acid	Teleapque			
Meglumine ioglycamate	Biligram			Cholecystography

Contrast Radiography of the Alimentary Tract

Indications

- Obstruction of the alimentary tract such as non radio opaque foreign bodies, tumour masses, stenosis of the tract etc
- Distortion of the wall of the alimentary tract like esophageal dilatations, stomach enlargement due to pyloric stenosis etc.
- Lesions in the wall of the alimentary tract like neoplacia, ulcers etc.
- Displacement of the alimentary tract due to presence of intrabdominal masses, ruptured diaphragm etc.

Contrast agents

Specially prepared colloidal barium sulphate is used routinely :

1. Dry powder: to be mixed with water (micropaque powder)
2. A prepared suspension in water usually 100 w/v, barium meal (micropaque) is used.
3. A paste of increased viscosity used to outline esophageal mucosa.

In cases where perforation of alimentary tract is suspected, it is advised to substitute barium with any organic iodine compound; Meglumine diatrizoate, which gets absorbed and excreted in cases of any extravasations.

Preparation of patient

Withhold food and water for 24 hours and if necessary enema is given. Small amounts of barium are given in such patients who are dehydrated. Use of General Anesthesia/sedation should be avoided as they can slow/arrest the passage of contrast agent and they may relieve and prevent the recognition of any nervous spasms or constriction of the tract.

A straight radiograph (one taken before the administration of the contrast agent") of abdomen should be taken before administration of barium sulphate. So that abdominal organs can be identified and opacities within could be demonstrated.

Quantity: 15-60 ml of 25-100% suspension.

Radiographs

- Taken immediately after administration
- Subsequent radiographs are taken at 15 to 60 minutes interval depending on the part of the tract and rate at which barium is moving. Both lateral and VD projections must be taken.
- In case of neoplasms, ulcers and other lesions, bowel should be emptied by starving, laxatives/enema. It has to be confirmed by taking preliminary radiographs.

Oesophagus

Patient Preparation is not necessary. Unless gross lesions are present, barium will pass through rapidly, to outline the organ radiographically, a very thick mixture of barium sulphate is administered. This will give thick streak of barium indicating the position of oesophagus in the chest (fig.78). It is done to detect abnormalities like Esophageal obstruction, stenosis, diverticulam, perforation, megaesophagus and mucosal disease. Oesophagus is normal without obstruction, if linear streaks are seen and barium meal quickly cleared in to the stomach. Barium gets accumulated cranial to obstruction site detecting the abnormality. If Esophageal outpouch filled with contrasts agent is noticed is suggestive of Diverticulam. (fig.79 & 80)

Stomach

Technique

1) Positive contrast radiography

Contrast media Micropaque (100% W/V Diluted) 5ml/kg body Weight. Barium Swallow (70% W/V Solution of barium sulphate 25 - 30ml/kg) is fed orally. To allow the movement of the barium into the duodenum and to concentrate it on the cardiac end of the stomach, the animal is first placed on its left side down or on its back and radiographed.

Then patient is placed upright or on its right side to outline the pyloric end. Barium normally passes into duodenum, but a nervous dog will retain the medium in the stomach and gives a false impression of a pyloric obstruction unless the examination is repeated.

After allowing time for the passage of barium sulphate into the intestine, the stomach should be radiographed again to see the residue of barium sulphate, which is outlining the foreign body or deep gastric ulcers (fig. 81). Radiograph is taken at 15 Min, 30 Min, 1 Hr interval. Further radiographs should be taken at hourly intervals until the contrast agent reaches the colon, to known gastric empting time and Intestinal transit time.

Indications: Radiolucent foreign body, Neoplasia, Dilatation, Pyloric stenosis, Ulcer, etc.

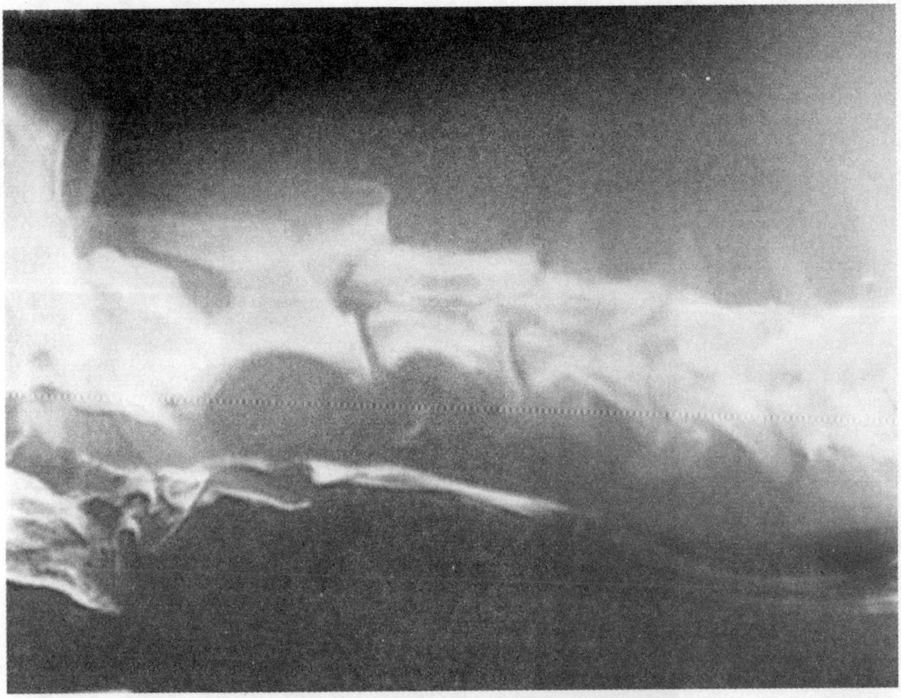

Fig. 78. Radiograph showing barium streak in oesophagus

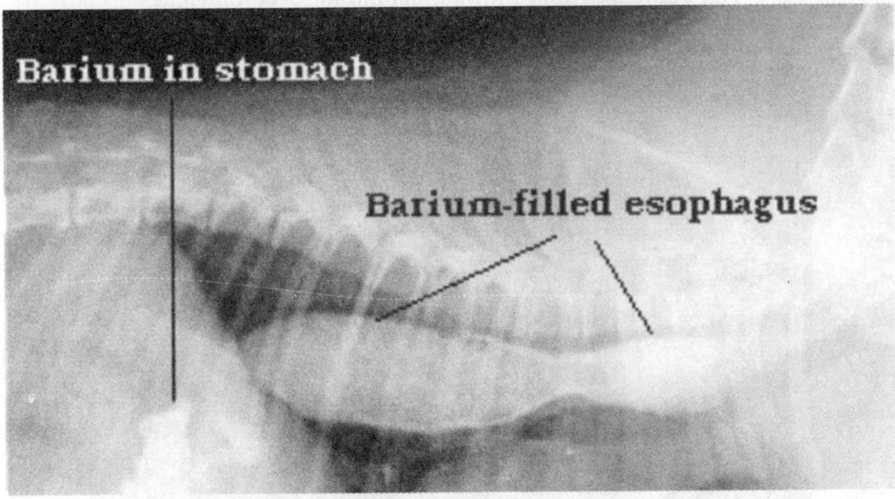

Fig. 79. Radiograph showing barium filled oesophagus indicating diverticulum (Lateral View)

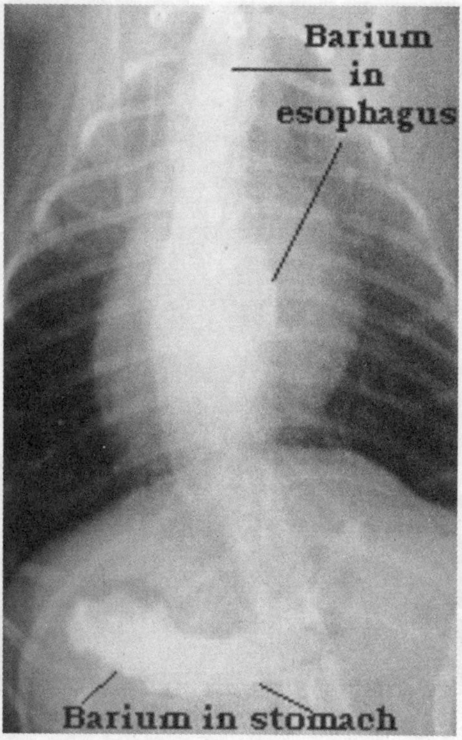

Fig. 80. Radiograph showing barium filled oesophagus indicating diverticulum (Ventrodorsal View)

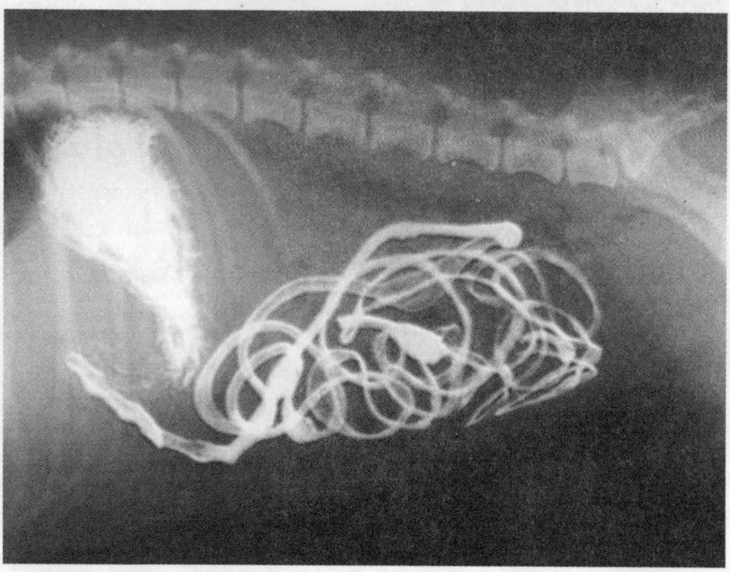

Fig.81. Positive Contrast Radiography of Stomach and Intestine

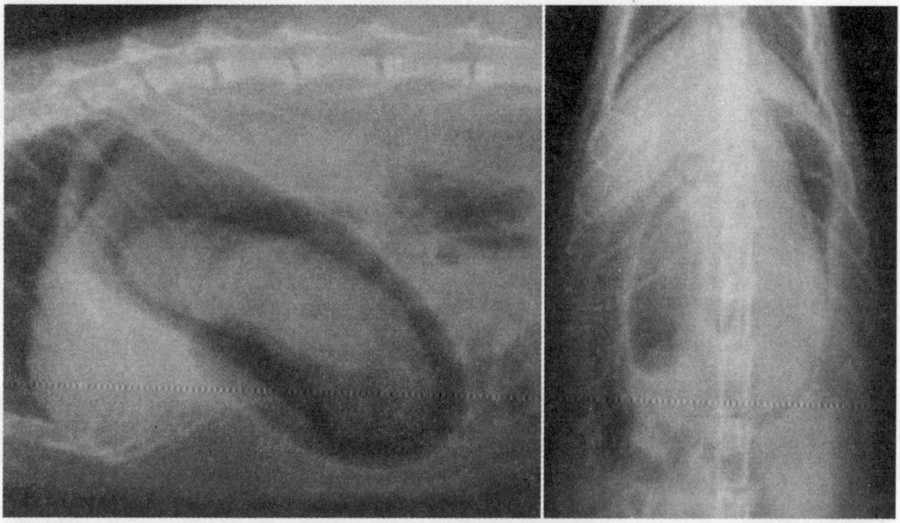

Fig.82. Double Contrast Radiography showing Gastrogram –Air (Lateral View & Ventrodorsal View)

2) Double contrast radiography

Administer of both positive contrast agent (micropaque or barium swallow) and negative contrast agents (air-10-15 ml/kg b. wt) via gastric intubation. Induction of gastric hypotonia by glucogon and addition of dimethicone as an antifoam agent to barium sulphate susp is done. Normal Gastric empting time 30 min to 3 hrs. If any delay in empting it suggested anomaly of stomach. If the clearance of contrast agent within 1 to 1.5 hr is seen then it is suggestive of gastritis. If spotting focally or diffused form is seen then it is suggestive of ulcers or abnormal growth. (fig.82)

Small intestine: barium 25% suspension

More dilute form is used for easy passage. Films at random may miss the outlining of significant lesions of bowel wall. It may show constriction due to peristalsis and gives a false impression of lesion. However consistent demonstration of identical lesion of the bowel wall in a series of radiographs would be of significance. (fig. 83 & 84)

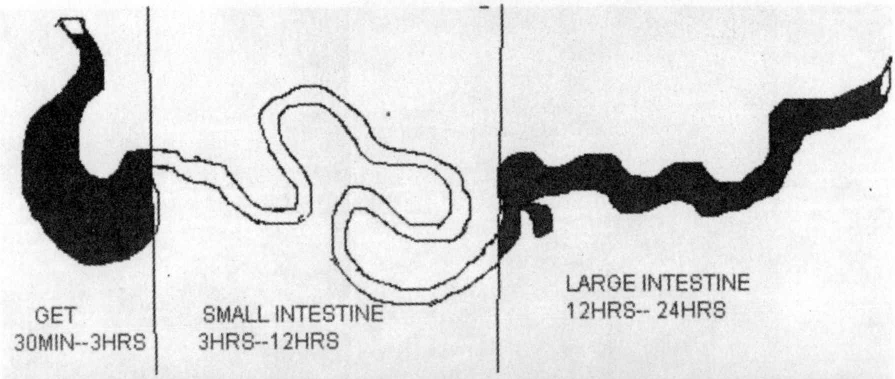

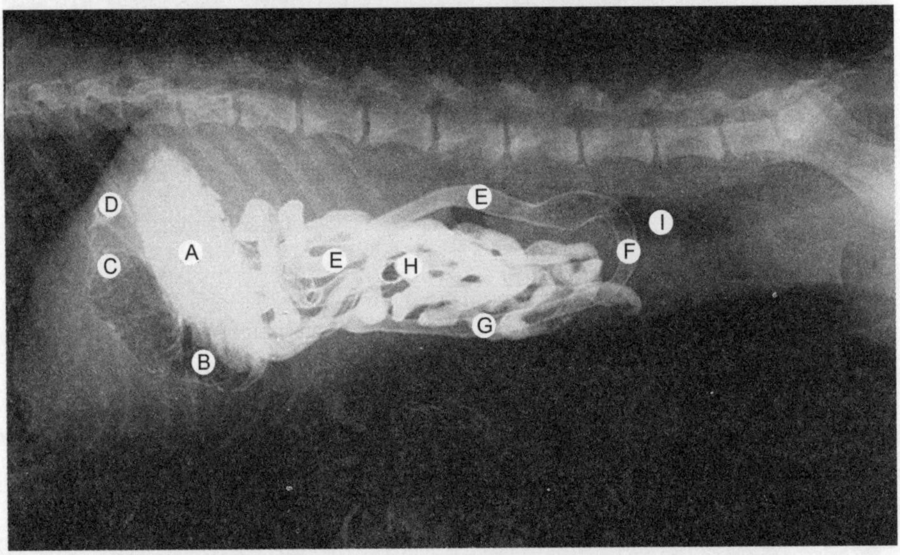

Fig.83. Lateral View: Abdomen - 1 hour after barium swallow

Stomach : A-Fundus B-Body; C-Pyloric Antrum; Duodenum D-Cranial Duodenal Flexure; E-Descending Duodenum; F-Caudal Duodenal flexure (Transverse Duodenum); G-Ascending Duodenum; H-Jejunal Loops; I-Descending Colon.

Large intestine

Barium enema is done by means of irrigation or enema by elevating hindquarter under general anesthesia to diagnose conditions like Megacolon, ulcerative colitis, fistula, intraluminal or extraluminal obstructions by taking subsequently radiographs (fig. 85)

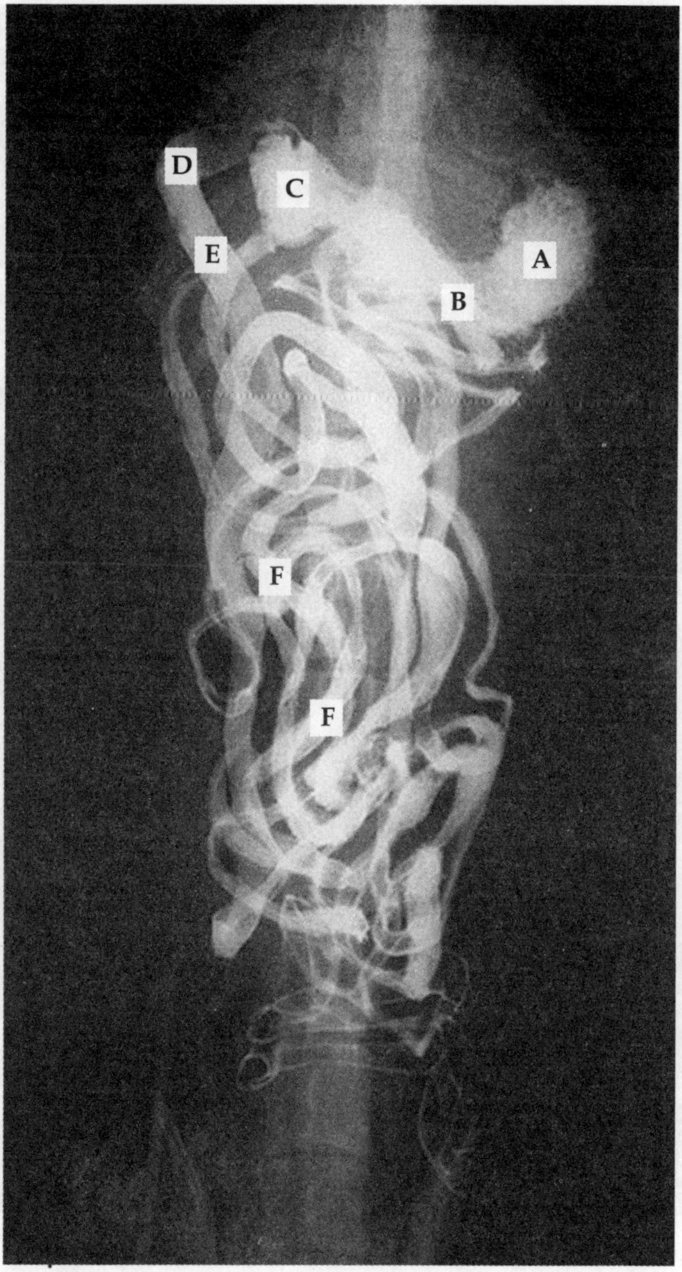

Fig.84. Ventrodorsal View: Abdomen - 1 hour after barium swallow

A. Fundus of the Stomach Body B. Gastric Body

C. Pyloric Antrum D. Cranial Duodenal Flexure

E. Descending Duodenum F. Jejunum

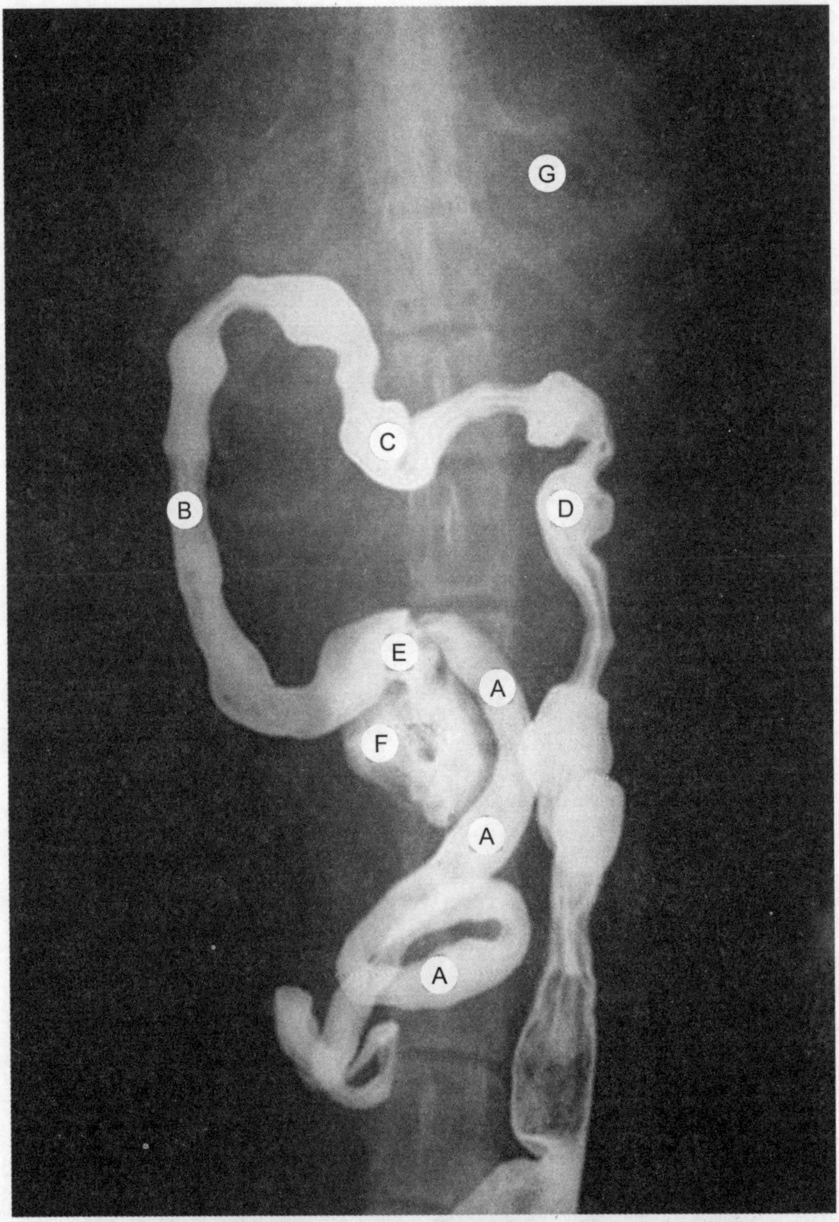

Fig.85. Ventrodorsal View: Abdomen – 3.5 hour after barium swallow

A. Ileum B. Ascending Colon

C. Transverse Colon D. Descending Colon

E. Site of Ileocolic and Cecocolic Orifices F. Cecum

G. Gas in Stomach

Double Contrast Radiography of Colon

Done using a balloon catheter air or carbon dioxide is injected at the rate of 11-30ml/kg in to the colon followed by barium enema- Barium sulphate 10-20% W/V is infused 1-1.5 ml/ kg b.wt. Triple contrast radiograph by-Pneumoperitonium. Radiographs are taken lateral and VD views. Double contrast enhances visualization of barium coated mucosal surface where as triple contrast helps clear demarcation of colonic wall.

Normal Colon looks like question mark (?) with smooth non-sacculated borders (fig. 86). Ceacum looks like coiled appearance in dog. Filling Defect indicates intraluminal masses Neoplasia, polyp, foreign body, intussusceptions. Abnormal Positioning of Colon can also be detected. If we find Mucosal irregularities, it indicates ulcers or inflammatory colitis.

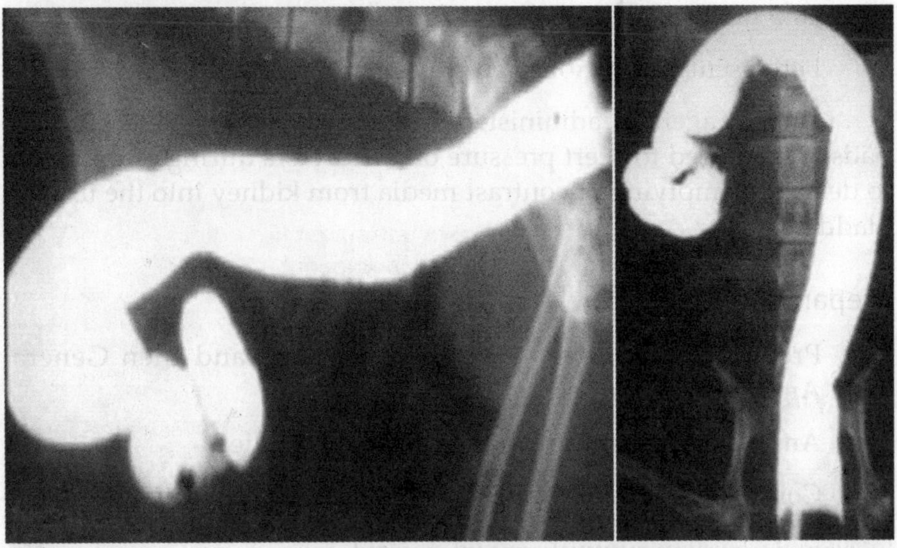

Fig.86. Positive Contrast (Barium Enema) of colon

Urography (Pyelography, Intravenous Pyelography, Excretory Urography)

Used to

- Increase the defination of kidney shadow when it cannot be identified in a plain radiograph.
- To show the presence/absence of lesions in kidney pelvis.

- To provide some indication of kidney function.
- To evaluate the size, shape and location of kidneys, ureter and urinary bladder.
- To know renal function test and urinary track patency.
- Diagnosis of nephroliths, tumor, uroliths, ectopic ureter, urethral rupture.

Contrast agents

Organic iodine compounds, after i/v administration are rapidly excreted through the urinary system

- 50% sodium diatrizoate (Hypaque)
- 70% sodium acetrizoate (dianosil-1ml/kg in small dogs)
- 60% Meglumine iothalamte-2ml/3kg-large dogs)

Perivascular injections can cause irritations.

Contrast agent is administered i/v; compression band and two pads are required to exert pressure on the ureters during examination to delay the emptying of contrast media from kidney into the urinary bladder.

Preparation of Patient

- Prepare the patient by giving an enema and then General Anesthesia.
- An abdominal compression bandage is applied
- Contrast agent is administered slow I/v over a period of 2-3 minutes.
- Radiographs are taken at 0,5,15 & 20th minute
- Compression bandage is removed and a radiograph is taken

Technique

Patient is placed in dorsal recumbency and a pressure band is applied and tightened (objective is to compress the ureters and obtain maximum concentration of the dye in the kidney. If not agent moves to the bladder and poor definition of renal pelvis will be seen). Slow i/v injection is made. Straight film is taken before injection and subsequent films at 0 min, 30sec, one min, 5 min and 20 minutes after completion of injection, radiographs are taken. Clinical application of this technique in veterinary practice is very limited, and there is a variation between the two kidneys in the amount of dye that is excreted. This technique is not used in patients where kidney function is altered or hampered (fig 87 & 88).

Alternative method

Using i/v transfusion of dilute form of contrast agent. In this case there will no necessity to withhold fluid or to compress the patients.

Normal Kidney: In Dog 2.5-3.5 times to the length of second lumbar vertebra,

In Cat 2.4-3.0 times to the length of second lumbar vertebra.

Abnormality

Small kidney: chronic pylonephritis, interstitial nephritis, hypo genesis infarction.

Large kidney: acute nephritis, subcapsular hematoma, and hydronephrosis, Neoplasia.

Extra renal contrast media: trauma, hydronephrosis (perforation)

Urethral abnormalities: dilation (hydroureter), ectopic ureter, rupture, neoplasia, Radiolucent calculi.

Cystography

- Diagnosis of small cystic calculi or Radiolucent calculi
- Determine location and integrity of bladder
- Chronic or recurrent lower urinary tract infection
- Assist in radiography of prostate gland

Techniques

- Positive contrast Cystography
- Pneumocystography
- Double contrast Cystography

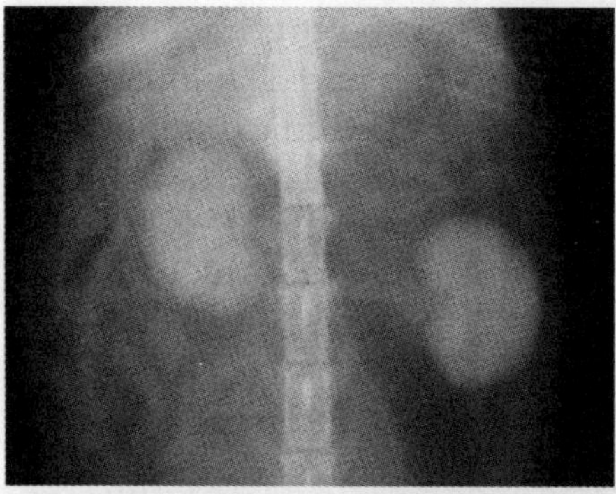

Fig.87. Nephrogram (5 min)

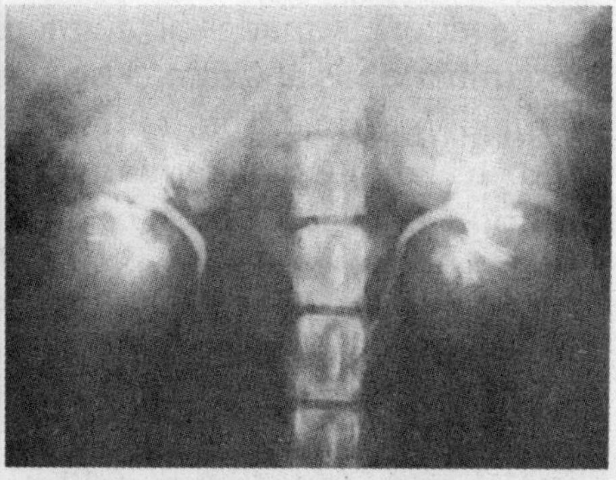

Fig.88. Pyelogram (20 min)

Contrast agents

1. ***Iodine compounds:*** 20% solution of sodium iodide in human beings. It can cause iodine hypersensitivity. Iodine preparations are useful in demonstrating the outline of urinary bladder, but they are likely to mask the presence of calculi.
2. *Air*: useful to demonstrate calculi
   Quantity: 40-100ml

Preparation of the patient

Animal is fasted and enema is done. Bladder is evacuated before examination. If possible blood clots or other deposit washed with sterile water or saline. Material is administered via the catheter into the bladder. Radiographs are taken immediately in both planes after completion of injection.

Positive Contrast Cystography

Introduce lubricated tip of urethral catheter in to the urethral opening and advance in to the bladder. Drain the urine from the bladder and lumen is flushed with normal saline once or twice. Introduce the water soluble contrast agent (sodium iothalamate 70% diluted to 10-20%) dogs 6-12 ml/kg. Radiographs are taken right lateral and ventrodorsal projections (fig.89).

Pneumocystography

Technique: Inflate the bladder with air 2-4ml /kg b wt. to desired level of distention. Radiographs are taken right lateral and ventrodorsal projections. (fig.90)

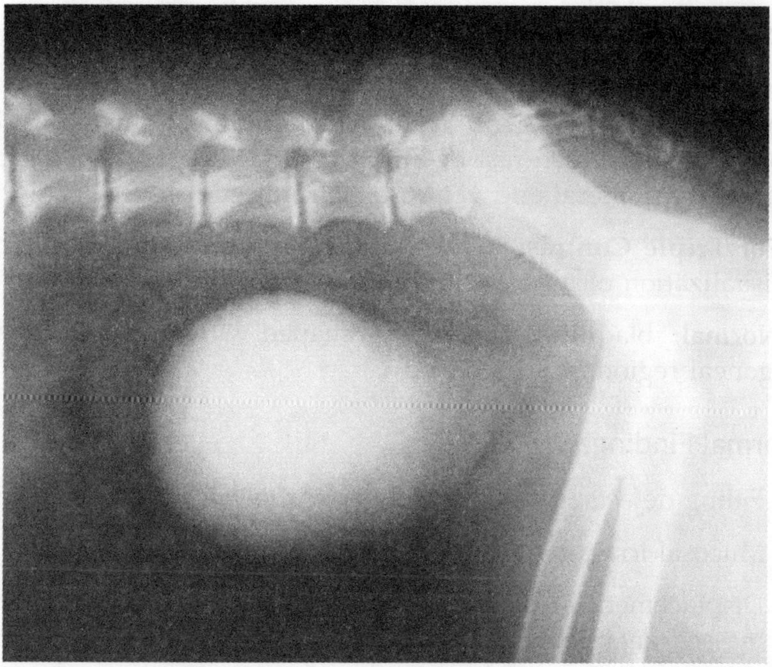

Fig.89. Positive Contrast Cystography in Dog

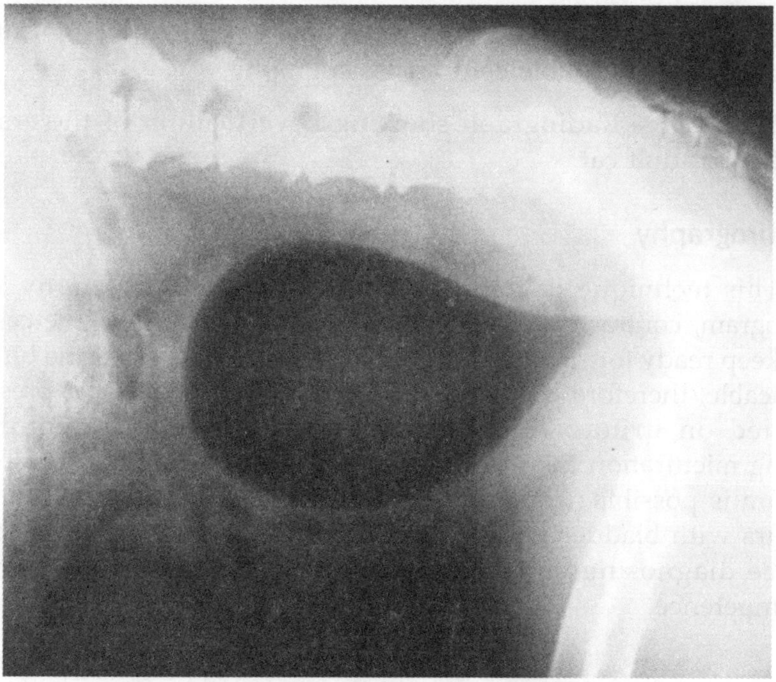

Fig.90. Pneumocystography in Dog

Double Contrast Radiography

Introduce air at 2-4ml/kg b wt followed by introducing 15-20 ml of positive Contrast Agent. Then roll the animal, this is to allow uniform coating of contrast agent on bladder Mucosa. Radiographs are taken right lateral and ventrodorsal projections. (fig.91).

For Triple Contrast -Create Pneumoperitonium It is enhances the visualization of mucosal and serosal wall surfaces.

Normal: -bladder is "tear drop" shaped with a smooth tapering at trigoneal region.

Abnormal Findings

- Filling defects: neoplasia, polyps, chronic cystitis, and calculi.
- Mucosal irregularities: neoplasia, inflammation.
- Displacement of bladder from its normal position: abdominal masses, enlargement of prostate.
- Extravasations of contrast: ruptured bladder.

Figure.92 - Transitional cell carcinoma of cranial bladder of cat demonstrated by double contrast Cystography.

Figure 93 - Radiograph showing Diverticulum of the cranial bladder of adult cat.

Urethrography

This technique is continuation of excretory urography after pyelogram, contrast material collected in bladder. Load the cassets and keep ready for radiographs. Wait for animal to pass urine but not applicable, therefore either by means of digital pressure or pressure applied on urinary bladder, Animal is forced to micturate, during micturation take 1or 2 radiographs by this demonstration of urethra is possible. (fig. 94). Radiograph (fig. 95) shows absence of urethra with bladder neck opening directly at the external urethral orifice diagnosing as congenital urethral sphincter mechanism incompetence.

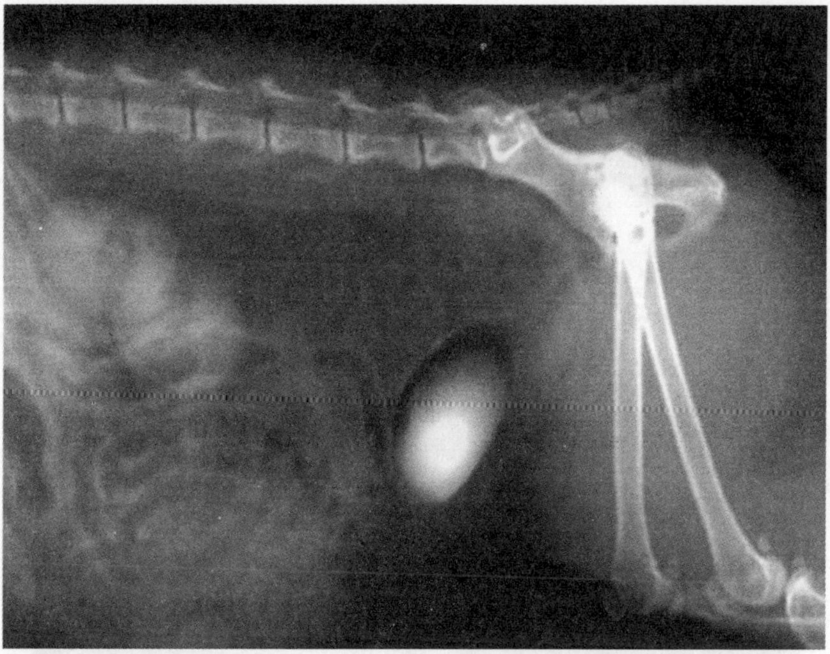

Fig.91. Double Contrast Cystography in Dog

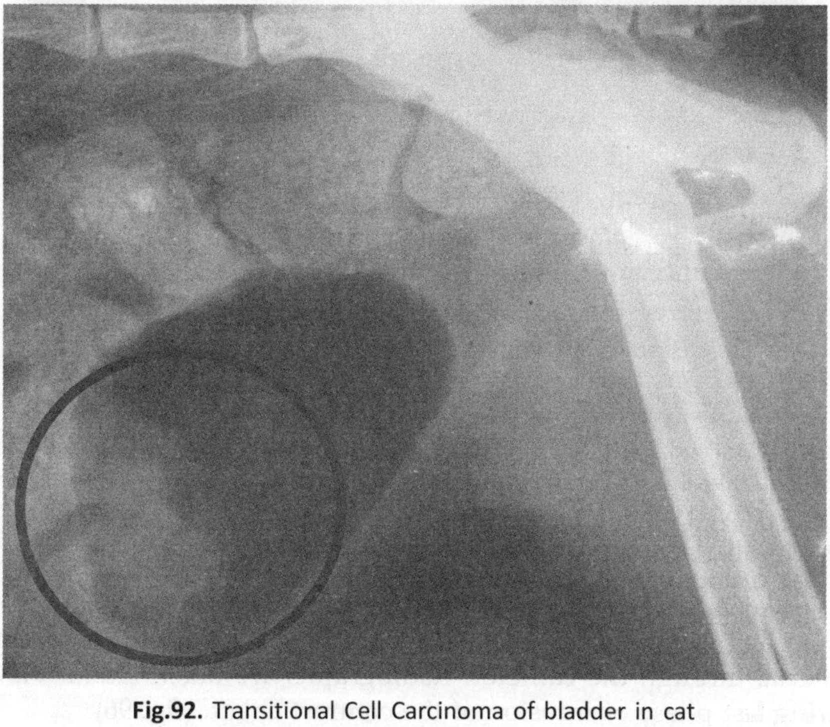

Fig.92. Transitional Cell Carcinoma of bladder in cat

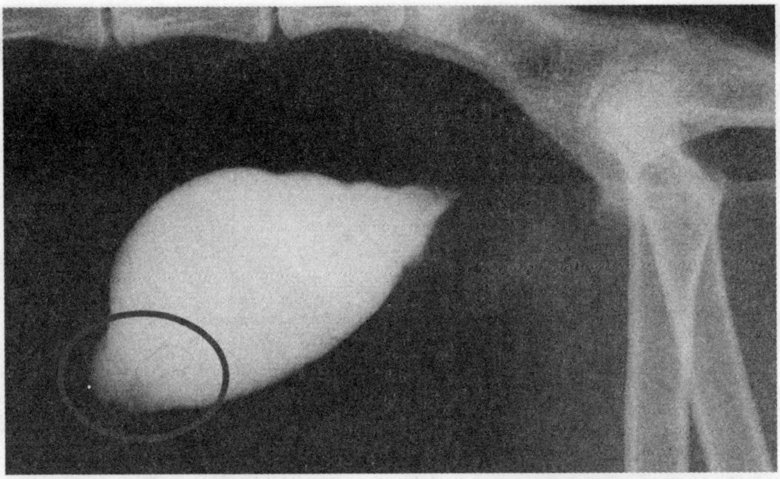

Fig.93. Radiograph showing Diverticulum of bladder in cat

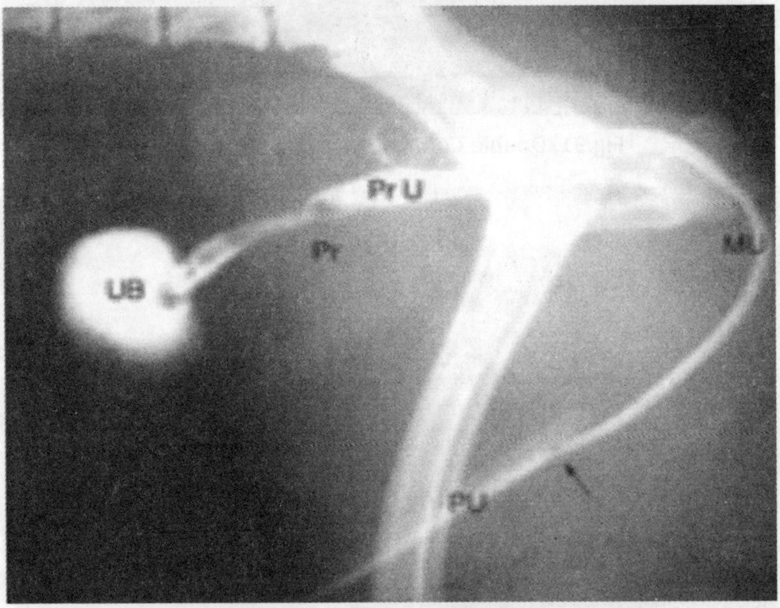

Fig.94. Urethrography (Male). PU - Penile urethra, MU - Membranous urethra. Pr U - Prastatic urethra, Pr – Prostate, UB - Urinary bladder

Retrograde Urethrography

Take catheter and insert in to the urethra for a short distance through urethral opening. Infuse about 2-3ml organic iodine contrast material through the catheter. Radiographs are taken lateral views during last phase of infusion of the contrast agent. (fig. 96).

Abnormal urethral findings

1. Filling defects: neoplasia, calculi, granuloma, blood clots.
2. Mucosal irregularities: adherence of contrast agent (lacerations, inflammation).
3. Extravasations of contrast material: urethral rupture. (fig.97).

Figure 98 - Penile urethral stricture following urethral obstruction the penile is very narrow and contrast medium filling a pre stricture urethral dilatation(d).

Figure 99 - Prostatic carcinoma (cat) - grass spillage of contrast medium in to the gland (arrowed) and irregularity of the urethra cranial to the gland associated with tumour invasion.

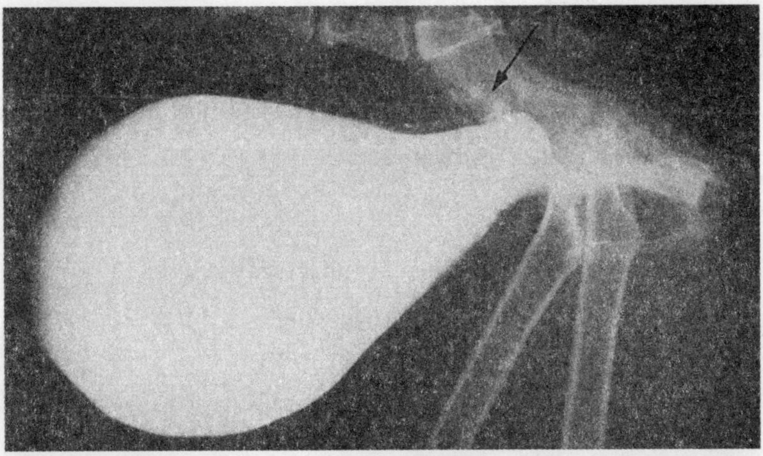

Fig.95. Congenital urethral sphincter incompetence

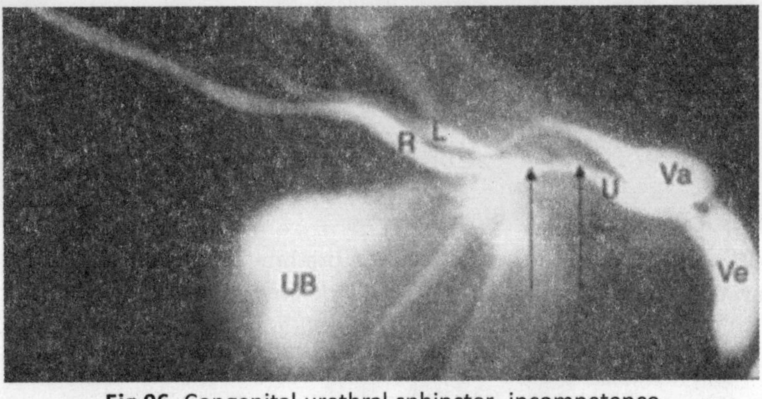

Fig.96. Congenital urethral sphincter incompetence
Bilateral Ectopic Ureters Ve-Vestibule, Va - Vagina, U-Urethra, UB-Urinary bladder, R-Right ureter, L-Left ureter

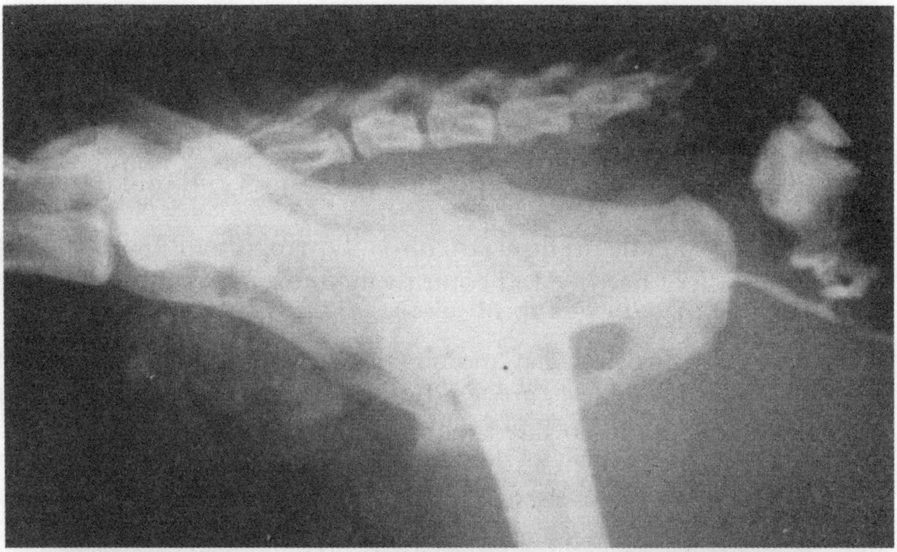

Fig.97. Extravasations of contrast material indicating urethral rupture

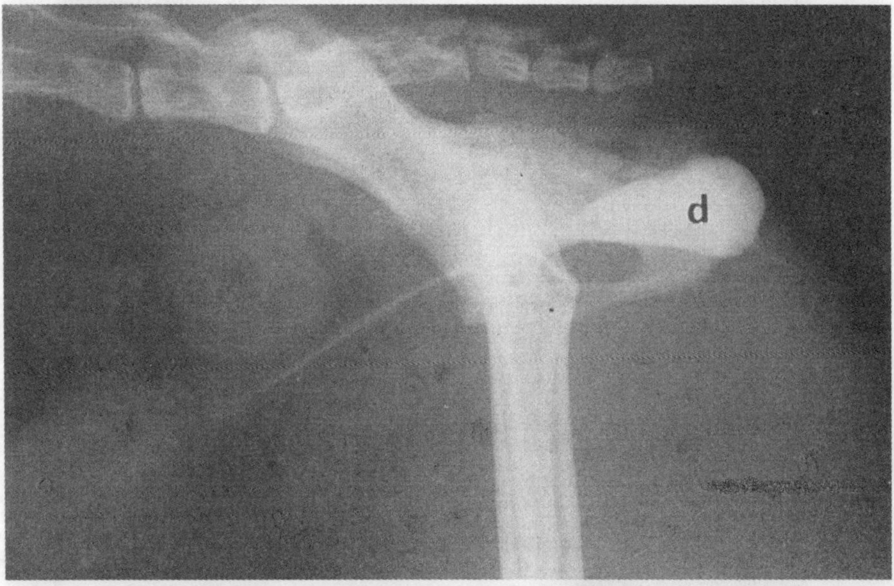

Fig. 98. Penile urethral stricture following urethral obstruction the penile is very narrow and contrast medium filling a pre stricture urethral dilatation(d).

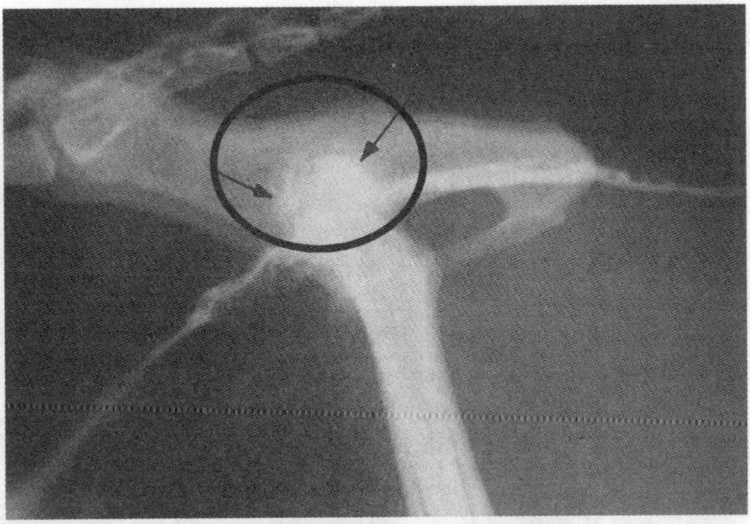

Figure 99. Prostatic carcinoma (cat)

Bronchography

Indications - For outlining and demonstration of bronchial tree, Investigation of chronic respiratory disease. Bronchial tumors, bronchectosis and displacement of pulmonary lobes.

Agent: oily or aqueous preparation of propyliodone (dianosil oily or dionosil aqueous)

Quantity: 5-30ml depending on the diameter of trachea and size of the animal.

Technique

Under General Anesthesia, animal is positioned on the sides with the lung under investigation downward. Then the contrast agent is administered into the trachea and allowed to spread allover the dependent bronchial tree. Lateral radiographs are taken after 3 minutes. Then the animal is brought to sternal recumbency and DV projection is taken.

Once radiography is complete, the dog is positioned so that the lung, which has filled, is uppermost and the chest is percussed to stimulate coughing. Most of the coughed up material is swallowed. In this technique, only one lung can be examined at a time and to repeat the procedure on the other side a gap of 48 hours is necessary (fig.100).

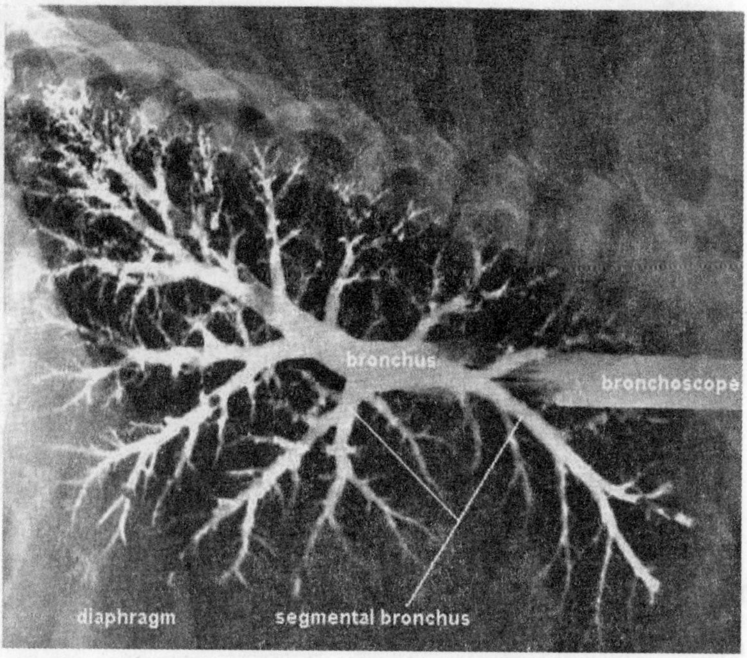

Fig. 100. Bronchography

Myelography

It is defined as radiographic examination of the spinal cord after introduction of contrast material into the sub arachnoids space.

Indications-spondilosis, IVD discontinuation or protrusion, chronic neck pain, lumbar pain, peresis, paralysis, paraplegia, intraspinal lesions, Spinal lesions,Vertebral canal hemorrhage, Spinal cord edema.

Contraindications: Meningitis, Myelomalacia, Recent use of phenothiazine tranquilizer or neuroleptic agents.

Agent

Agent must be non-irritant

1. Neo-hydriol fluid: oily fluid containing 40% iodine in organic combination
2. Myodil: mixture of isomeric ethyl iodophenylundecylate containing 30% organically combined iodine

   Quantity: 0.5 to 2 ml

Technique

Spinal needle of 19g to 21g, 3 to 3/12" length is used. Light General Anesthesia, back of the head should be clipped and shaved. Injection is usually made into the sub arachnoids space at cisterna magna. The position of the needle in the cisterna magna is confirmed by dripping of cerebrospinal fluid (CSF) from the needle. Introduce spinal needle with a stylet in to the subarachnoid space through foramen magnum. Calculate dose of Metrizamide 0.3-0.4ml/kg b wt. then attach a syringe to the needle and aspirate CSF in equal quantity of contrast material to be injected. Then the contrast agent is slowly injected, about 5 minute over the whole injection.

Head must be kept slightly raised to prevent passage of material into the skull. Radiographs are taken in the lateral plane by directing the x-ray beam horizontally and having the film held in stand against the side of the animal. Radiographs in lateral and VD position are taken as soon as possible and at 5, 10, 15, 30 minutes (fig. 101).

CERVICAL >>>THORASIC >>>LUMBAR "SACRAL

(0-5min) >>>>> (5-15min) >>>>>(15–30min)

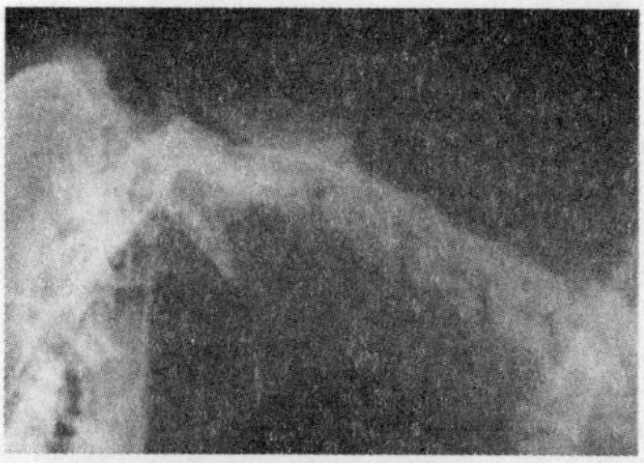

Cervicalregion

Thoracicregion

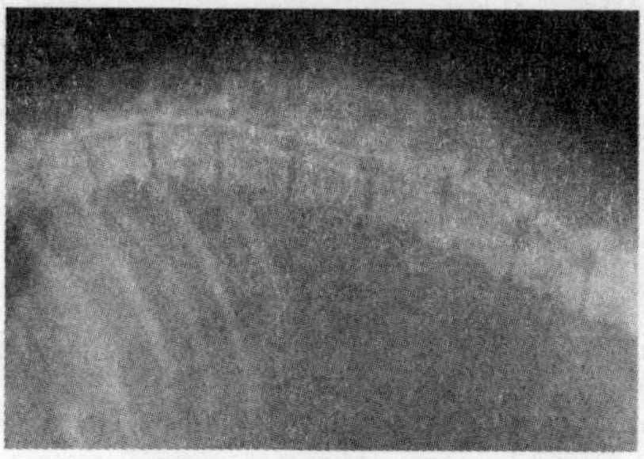

Thoraco-Lumbar Region

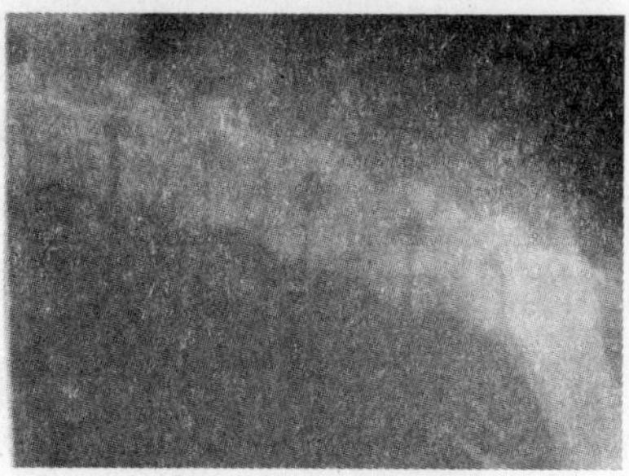

Lumbar Region

Fig. 101. Myelography

There are certain disadvantages with these agents

- They are oily and hence do not mix with CSF. They tend to globulate and pass slowly along the spinal canal. They get absorbed slowly, hence remain in the spinal canal for indefinite periods.
- There is definite risk of damaging the CNS during injection.

Angiography

It is the radiographic demonstration of certain areas of the vascular system by the injection of water-soluble organic compounds into a suitable blood vessel.

1. Arteriography	Artery
2. Venography	Vein
3. Portal venography	Portal venous system
4. Aortography	Aorta
5. Angiocardiography	Heart
6. Cerebral angiography	Brain

Indications

- For the demonstration of occlusion of a particular blood vessel by internal thrombus or external pressure.
- To show anatomical variation or pathological lesions of vascular system.
- To provide evidence of inaccessible neoplasm (usually within the brain) by demonstrating the abnormalities of usual vascular pattern of the patient.

Contrast agents

Waters soluble organic iodine compounds eg: dioginal, hypaque-Bayers.

Technique

Injection is made into a blood vessel. Exposures are to be made immediately after the injection. Multiple exposures are made after each injection of bolus dose. Procedure is done under General Anesthesia.

Arteriography

Indications: To study the arterial pattern in normal subjects from anatomy point of view and to study variations in patterns due to a pathological process. It is also indicated to diagnose arterial occlusion.

1. Femoral region	External iliac
2. Metatarsal region	Tibial or cranial
3. Hind digit	Dorsal metatarsal
4. Fore digit	Dorsal Metacarpal
5. Metacarpal region	Median
6. Cerebral angiography	Common carotid artery
7. Abdominal arteriography	Common carotid artery or Femoral artery

Technique: Anaesthetise the animal, Expose the desired vessel and catheterize. Inject contrast material using appropriate dose (Approximately 10-30 ml in calf, 2-8 ml in dog sodium iothalamate (70%w/v). Take radiograph during the last phase of the injection (fig. 102 to 104).

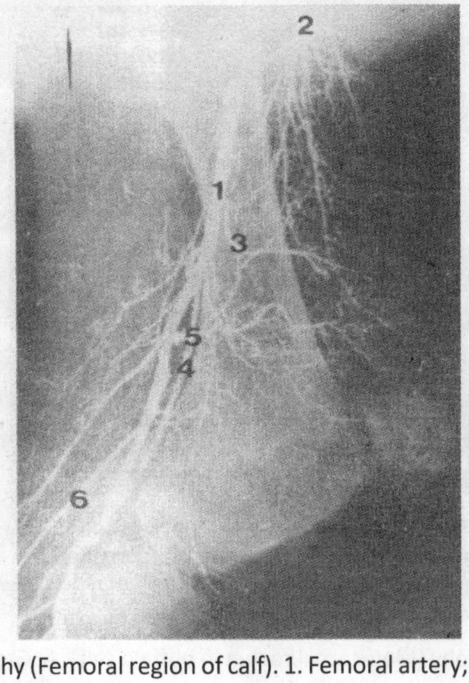

Fig.102. Arteriography (Femoral region of calf). 1. Femoral artery; 2. Lateral circumflex iliac artery; 3. Descending genicular artery; 4. Saphenous artery; 5. Nutrient artery; 6. Caudal femoral artery

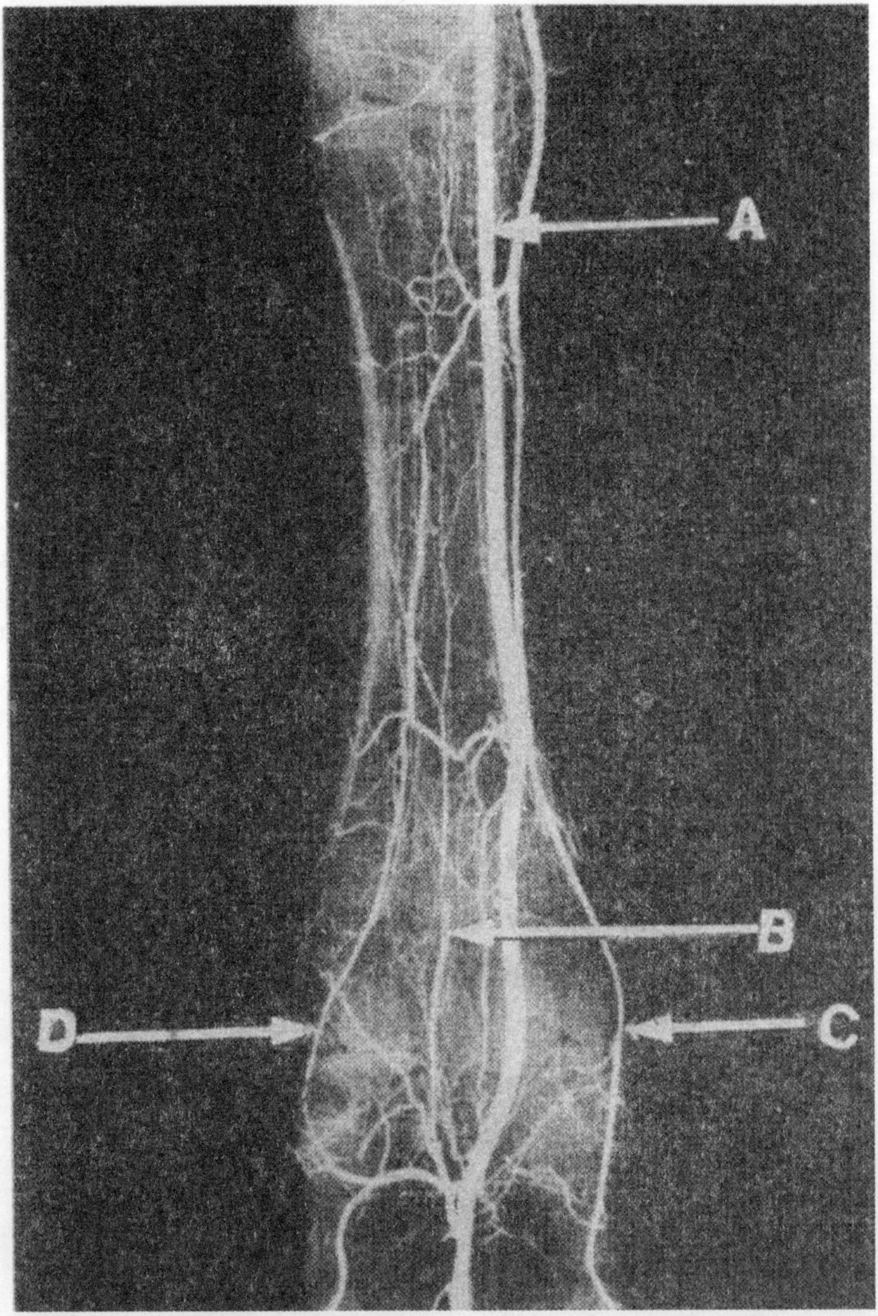

Fig.103. Arteriography (Metacarpal region in buffalo calf). A. Great metacarpal artery; B. Dorsal metacarpal artery; C.Medial palmar metacarpal artery; D. lateralpalmar metacarpal artery

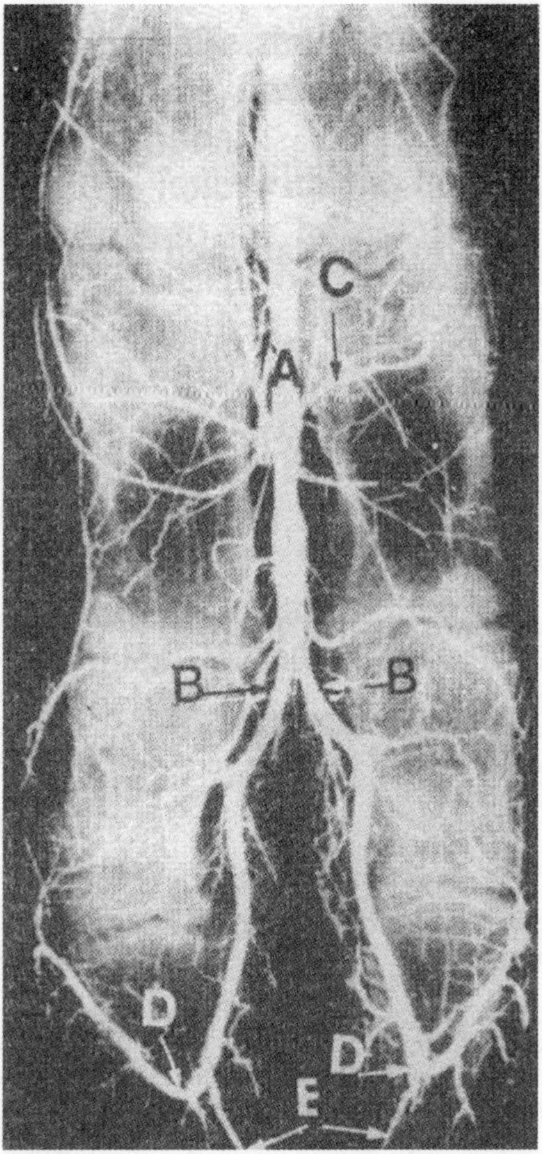

Fig.104. Arteriography (Bovine digital region of foot)

Angiocardiography

1. Used for demonstration of congenital or acquired lesions of the heart.
2. To study the **size** and **shape** of heart, its chambers and its vessels.
3. Detect cardiac abnormalities (right to left shunt, valvular disease).

4. Demonstrate filling defect.
5. To detect cardiomyopathies.
6. Identification of intracardiac thrombi.
7. Evaluation of aorta, anterior and posterior venacava to rule out occlution, Emboli, stricture.
8. To obtain satisfactory concentration of dye within the heart, which is achieved by injecting the contrast agent through a catheter introduced into jugular vein and passed along anterior venecava until it, reaches the right atrium.

Dorso palmar aspect

A. Common digital artery
B. Digital arteries
C. Distal palmar arch
D. Terminal arches
E. Laminar vessels

Angiocardiogarms demonstrating the chambers of right side of the heart is made by simply injecting contrast agent directly into jugular vein and taking a single lateral radiograph of heart immediately upon completion of the injection. Left ventricle and aorta have been visualized by cardiac puncture and direct injection of dye into the left ventricle.

Technique

1. Selective Type : Contrast material is directly deposited in to the organ or structure (ex: heart) with the help of angiographic catheter.
2. Non-Selective Type : The Contrast agent is injected in main trunks of vessels like aorta/venacava and get distributed in the focused structure.

Catheter is placed in the closest accessible vessel to the heart in order to reduce resistance to bolus injection. Jugular vein is preferred but may be cephalic or saphenous veins also tried. Contrast agent a warm to body temperature to reduce viscosity and to minimize animal discomfort. Dose 400-450mg I/kg b.wt. This dosage can be repeated up to three times of a total dose of 1300mg I/kg b.wt. Take radiographs as rapidly as possible that is ventro-dorsal and left lateral position (fig. 105).

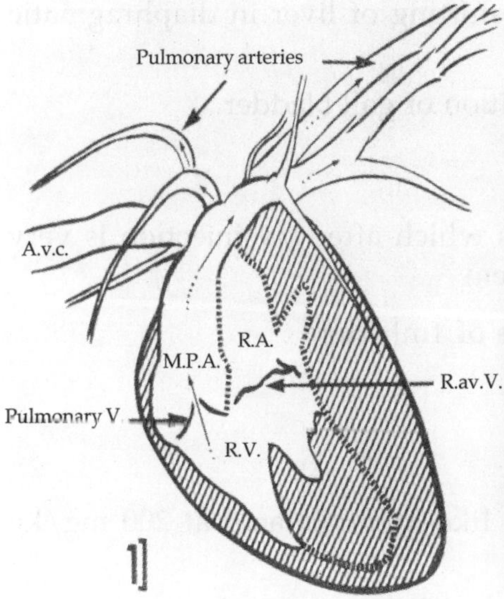

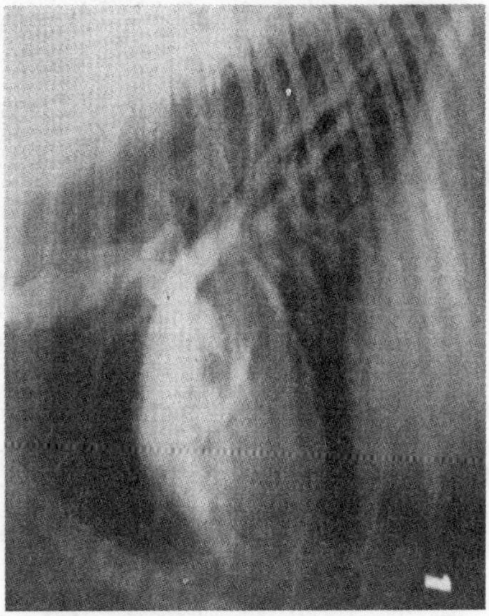

Fig. 105. Angiocardiography

Normal Positive contrast transit times through the heart

Animal	Transit Time (sec)
Cat	6-8
Small dog	6-8
Medium dog	7-9
Large dog	7-10

Cerebro-angiography

Procedure is designed to visualize the arterial supply to the brain and also used to demonstrate variations from the normal vascular pattern associated with the neoplacia and other lesions. The upper portion of the common carotid artery is exposed surgically, 5-7 ml of contrast agent (Hypaque) is injected into this after temporary occlusion of the external carotid artery (order to shunt the contrast agent into the internal carotid circulation). Again a rapid film-changing device is advantageous. One exposure at 2-3 seconds after injection and another at 6 seconds should be done.

Cholecystography

Indications

- It is useful in detecting radiolucent gallstones.

- Locating of gall bladder in shifting of liver in diaphragmatic hernia.
- To know the anatomical position of gall bladder.

Contrast agent

Biligrafin- iodine compounds which after i/v injection is very largely excreted to the biliary system

Dose: 30% solution at the rate of 1ml/2kg.

Preparation of the patient

ORAL CHOLECYSTOGRAPHY

- Feed oral cholecystopaques like Iopanoic acid at 200 mg/kg b wt.
- The radiographs were taken at different intervals
- The relative radiopacity and size of the bladder increased progressively from 10hr onwards up to 40 hr and was maximum from 20-30 hr intervals.
- After 30 hr the radiopacity and size of the bladder starts decreasing thereafter and the bladder shadow completely disappears at 60hr interval.

Intravenous Cholecystography

Food and water is withheld for 12 hours prior to the injection of the dye. General Anesthesia is done. Contrast agent is administered by slow i/v injection over 3 minutes time. Lateral radiograph of anterior abdomen is taken centering dorsal and slightly anterior to xiphid sternum. Radiographs are taken immediately before injection of the drug and 20-30 minutes and 90 minutes after administration.

Normal: The gallbladder extends from 8th –11th rib depending upon its fullness (fig.106).

Abnormal: Filling Defect indicates gallstones even can diagnose Abnormal position of gallbladder.

Peritoneography

1. Pneumoperitoneography
2. Doublecontrastperitoneography

Indications

- To visualize the outlines of various abdominal organs.
- To locate suspected abdominal masses.

Contrast agent

Air or oxygen, amount 200-1000 ml depending on the size of the animal.

Preparation: routine fasting and emptying and often General anesthesia is used.

PNEUMOPERITONEOGRAPHY

Technique: Insert a 5cm long 14-16 G needle (18G in a dog) attached to a catheter into the peritoneal cavity i,e left paralumbar fossa. slowly infuse CO_2, O_2 or compressed air till abdomen is moderately distended. Avoid over inflation. Withdraw the needle. Obtain standing left and right lateral radiographs. In small ruminants and dogs, Ventro-dorsal projections can also be obtained.

Double Contrast Peritoneography

Technique: Infuse a water-soluble positive contrast agent in the peritoneal cavity (e.g. sodium iothalamate 70% W/V @ 0.5 ml/kg). Create Pneumoperitonium as described for pneumoperitoneography. Roll from side to side to ensure uniform distribution of the contrast agent into the peritoneal cavity. Obtain standing right & left lateral projections. In small ruminants and dogs, VD projections are also obtained. (fig.107).

Sialography

i) To diagnose space occupying lesions of the parotid gland

ii) To locate the site of obstruction in the stenson's duct

iii) To locate the site of leakage of saliva in case of sialocele.

iv) Useful in demonstrating salivary calculi and fistula.

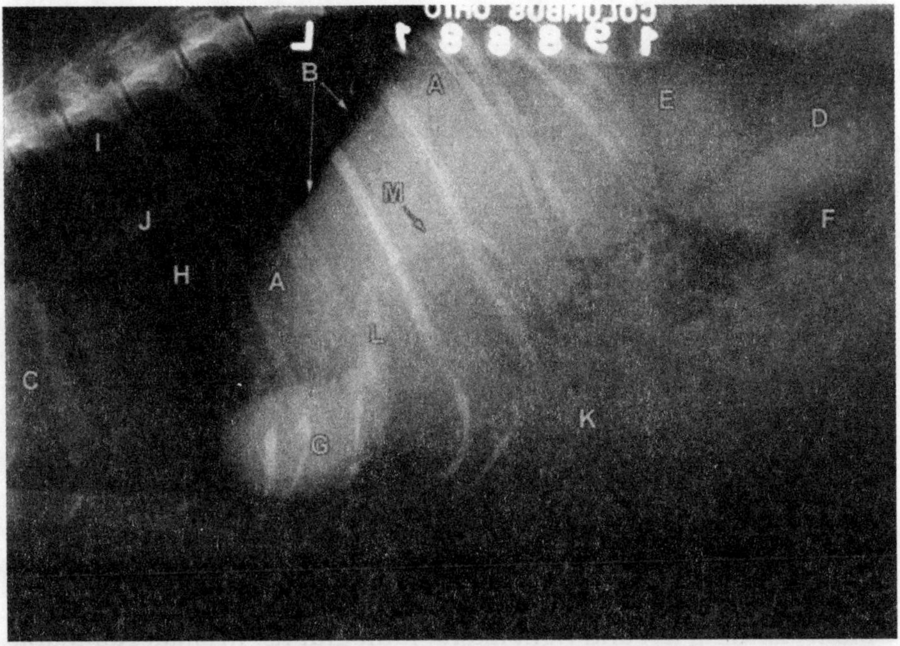

Fig.106. Cholecystography. A- Liver; B- Diaphragm; C- Heart; D- Left kidney; E- Right kidney; F- Descending colon; G-Gall bladder; H- Caudal venecava; I- Descending aorta; J- Pulmonary vessels; K- Jejunal loops; L- Cystic duct; M-Bile duct

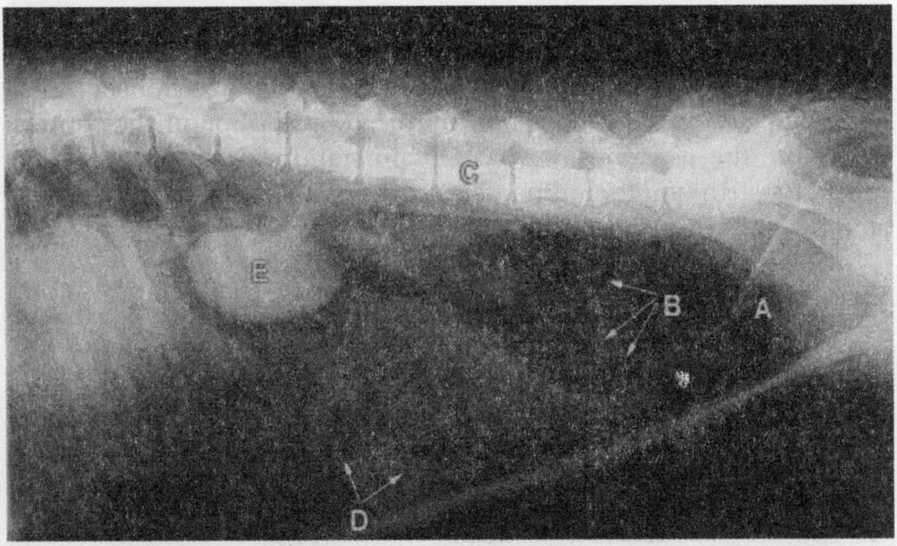

Fig.107. Peritoneography. A-Descending Colon; B-Gas in Small Intestine; C-L4; D-Cecum; E-Right Kidney

Technique

1. Retrograde: directly in to salivary duct

Cannulate the salivary duct through its opening in the oral cavity, in Cat-it opens at upper 2nd cheek tooth and in Dog-it opens at upper 3rd cheek tooth. Secure the cannula tightly by a ligature to prevent backflow of the contrast agent. Infuse 3-6 ml of water-soluble contrast agent and obtain a lateral projection at the end of injection.

2. Ante grade: injection of contrast material directly in to salivary gland

Injection of water-soluble contrast agent is directly infused into the glandular tissue and serial radiographs are taken. Any agent which decreases the flow of saliva e.g., Atropine, should not be administered before sialography.

Arthrography

Techniques

1. Negative contrast Arthrography
2. By using positive contrast agent
3. Double contrast Arthrography

Positive Contrast Arthrography

Arthrography should be performed under General Anesthesia. Prepare small area over the joint and aseptic puncture using 19 gauge 1.5" disposable needle. Needle placement in the joint space can be verified by aspiration of synovial fluid. Inject the contrast material followed by joint is manipulation. Radiographs are taken in Mediolateral & Posterioanterior plane.

Double Contrast Arthrography

Using aseptic technique, insert 19G hypodermic needle into joint. Remove as much synovial fluid as possible. Inject 2-3ml of water-soluble iodine based contrast agent and 10-15ml of air in to the joint. Flex and extend the joint several times. Then take radiographs in Anterioposterior, Posteroanterior, Mediolateral, Lateromedial and oblique projections.

Fasciagraphy

It is a contrast radiographic study of tendons and associated structures. This procedure is indicated to diagnose Adhesions, Calcification and Rupture of tendon and muscles.

Technique: Sedate the animal in lateral recumbency with the limb to be examined uppermost. Apply a tourniquet each proximal and distal to the site. Introduce a 16-18 G needle, using aseptic technique, between the muscle and tendon. Attach the three-way stopcock and a 50ml glass syringe to the needle. Inject room air till area between the two tourniquets is moderately distended then remove the needle. Obtain lateral projection Radiographs. Remove air and then tourniquets after the procedure.

Sinography

Technique: Preliminarily plain radiograph should be taken it may show cause of sinus (ex. foreign body or infection of adjacent bone) or presence of gas shadow. Contrast agents commonly used to outline the sinus tracks are the oily preparations since these are not irritating and they are not easily absorbed and removed from the site easily. First remove the discharge from the sinus track and irrigate one or two times by using normal saline. Then contrast agent is introduced as far as possible in to the cavity, by using a syringe along with narrow nozzle. Finally any contrast agent split on to the skin should be carefully removed before taking radiographs. Take radiographs in different views.

Renal Angiography

The technique is used to visualize renal vascular architecture and also helps to assess renal cortex-to-medulla ratio.

Technique: Using aseptic precautions expose and catheterize the femoral artery with a radiopaque catheter. Under fluoroscopic guidance, advance the catheter into the renal artery through abdominal aorta. Infuse small test dose of water-soluble iodine based contrast agent to confirm placement of the catheter. Infuse contrast agent (e.g. sodium iothalamate 70% W/V @ 0.5 to 1.0 ml/5kg). Obtain serial radiographs during last phase of injection and immediately after completion of infusion. (fig.108).

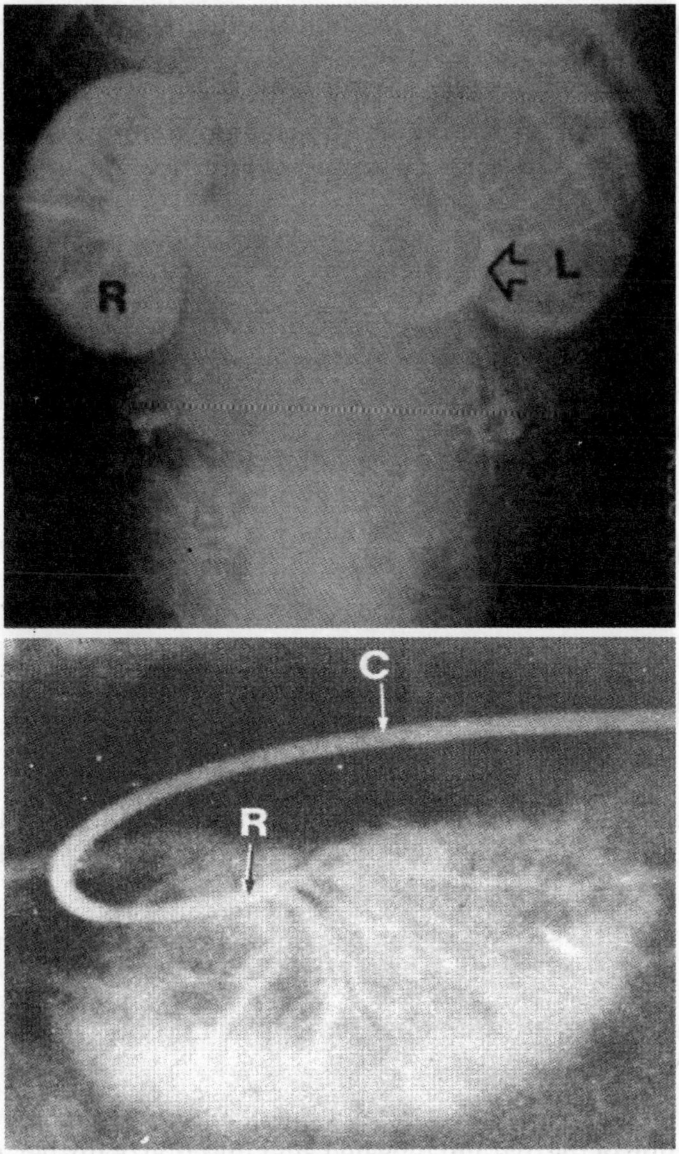

Fig- 108. Renal Angiography

Left kidney of goat C-catheter R-main Renal artery

Osteomedullography / Intraosseous Phlebography

The technique is used to visualize and extraosseous venous channels of a long bone. It can be used to aid diagnosis of Delayed and non-union of a fracture, Degenerative arthritis, bone neoplasm and even to diagnose avascular necrosis.

Technique: Anaesthetise the animal with the limb to be examined lowermost. Expose the distal metaphyseal end from the medial side using all aseptic precautions. Drill a hole with the help of an IMP pin in the metaphyseal region. Insert into the hole a 10cm long spinal needle. Ensure correct placement of the needle into the marrow cavity.

Demonstration of Sinus Tracts

Prior to radiography check for the presence of foreign bodies, clean the part remove as much discharge as possible. The dye Lipidol Lofay is introduced through a syringe and a blunt needle. Radiographs are taken in two planes.

Contrast radiography of the genital tract of the Bitch

Indications

- For outlining the uterus and uterine tubes and the ovaries
- To show the lesions of these structures which cannot be demonstrated in a plain radiograph.

Agent

Water soluble, permitting absorption and elimination from the uterus and comparatively viscous so that it does not spill from the uterus.

Eg, Viskidol Six and Skiodon sodium amount ranging from 1 to 6 ml

Contrast agent is administered into the uterus via the catheter (Metal bitch catheter)

Radiographs are taken in both the planes immediately after the introduction of the dye and repeated after injection of further amounts.

Lymphangiography: For demonstration of lymphatic system, involves the identification and surgical exposure of the lymphatic ducts of the fore and hind limbs and direct introduction of the agent Ethiodol. Radiographs are taken immediately.

27

Biological Effects of Radiation, Radiation Hazards and their Prevention by Adoption of Safety Measures

Biological effects

X-ray photon → cell → loss of electrons → atom which surplus positive charge → cell (high chemical reactivity)→ biological effects

Cell injury

- Physiological
- Pathological
- Radiation sickness

Radiation effect

- Somatic-to a person life time-leukemia, malignant tumors etc.
- Genetic-affects generations

Effects of radiation

a) **Direct**: due to absorption of radiant energy by molecules

b) **Indirect**: due to products of radiation decomposition (radiolysis) of water and other body solutions

H_2O → (H) +(OH) and free radicals

Adding oxygen by cells → H_2O_2 – a highly reactive and mutagenic causing biological damage.ie. Break in chemical bonds of proteins, nucleic acid and lipids

Damage to DNA molecule

Change of base, loss of base, and H^+ bond breakage between chains etc leads to biological effect. Pyramidines are more sensitive than purines of which thiamine is most sensitive. DNA damage alters the genetic information leading to mutations and disturbed cell proliferation.

Radiation sensitivity of different body cells

Radiation sensitivity refers to loss of reproductive capability of the proliferating cells. Hence cells, which regularly proliferate, seem to be more radiosensitive than cells that do not proliferate (nerve and muscle) which are radio resistant.

Order of increasing radio resistant/Order of decreasing radiosensitive

Lymphoid cells
↓
Epithelial cells of small intestine
↓
Haemopoitic cells
↓
Germinal cells
↓
Epithelial cells of skin
↓
Connective tissue cells
↓
Cartilage
↓
Growing bone cells
↓
Cells of brain
↓
Spinal cord
↓
Cells of skeletal muscle
↓
Mature bone

Species susceptibility

LD 50/30: dose of radiation that kills 50% of population within a period of 30 days

Rabbit
↓
Rat
↓
Mouse
↓
Hamster
↓
Guinea pig
↓
Man
↓
Dogs
↓
Pig
↓
Goat

Expressed in Gray (Gy), 1 Gy = 100 rads

Early Vs late radiation effects

Early effects. radiation sickness (Acute radiation syndrome).

	Supralethal dose 1000rads(10Gy)	**Medium lethal dose 500rads95Gy)**	**Sub lethal dose 200rads(2Gy)**
1st day	Nausea, vomition		
1st and 2nd week	Nausea, vomition, severe throat inflammation, dehydration, emaciation and even death		
3rd week		General malice, anorexia, haemorrhage, throat inflammation, emaciation and death	Loss of appetite, alopecia, haemorrhage and diarrhea

Radiation Injury to Tissues

a) **Lymphoid tissue**: Lymphocytes of Lymph Node, thymus and spleen are highly radiosensitive. Within 15 minutes after total body irradiation, lymphocytopenia and regeneration after 3 to 5 hours. It can cause organ shrinkage, formation of abscess, ulcers and haemorrhage

b) **Bone marrow**: Erythroblast are most sensitive, myelocytes are less sensitive.

c) **Cardiovascular system:** Heart, large arteries and veins are radio resistant. Endothelium of capillaries are most radiosensitive leading to capillary occlusion

d) **Digestive system**: most of the clinical signs are due to damage to the digestive system. Ulcers and erosions of buccal cavity. Pharynx and oesophagus are relatively radio resistant but high radiation dose may cause necrosis and sloughing

   Stomach: is radiosensitive it changes within 30 minutes

   Duodenum: most radiosensitive of the small intestine ***Large intestine***: less radiosensitive causes ulceration

e) **Skin**: radiation erythema –due to germinal epidermis damage. Maximum tolerable dose to skin is 10Gy.

f) **Respiratory system**: radiation causes pneumonitis

g) **Urinary system**: renal ischemia-hyper tension. Ureter and urinary bladder -relatively resistant

h) **Vision**: conjunctivitis, 3-10 Gy can induce cataract

i) **Male reproductive system**: male accessory organs, epididymis, vasdeferens –radioresistant 2-4Gy can cause sterility. Spermatozoa - radiosensitive

j) **Female reproductive system**: ovary, ova and granulose cells are radio-sensitive.

k) **Brain spinal cord, peripheral nerves, liver, gall bladder, bones, tendons and muscles**: are radio resistant.

Delayed effects

Effect is seen for several months in rats and mice. 10-20 months or years or seen more in humans which leads to Shortening of life span, leukemia, malignant tumors and cataracts.

Maximum Permissible Dose (MPD)

It is the level of exposure, which will not cause any observable symptoms of radiation damage. It is a level where no appreciable injury will be manifested in life of a person.

MPD for veterinarian and associated staff

	First use	One year
Whole body	100 m rem	5000 m rem
Hand, fore arm and leg	1500	75,000

Unit of measurement

(eV)

Electron volt measures the energy of an x ray expressed in thousand (KeV).

Roentgen (R)

Measures quantity of ionization (x ray and Gamma rays).

R is the quantity of x rays/Gamma radiation, which produces one electric unit in 1 cc of dry air at 0°C and 760mm Hg.

Rad (Radiation absorbed dose)

Unit of absorbed dose after any type of ionizing radiation.

One Rad = Radiation necessary to deposit energy of 100 ergs in 1 g irradiated material.

Rem (Roentgen equivalent man)

One rem = rad x quality factor.

Quality factor-Relates to the biological effectiveness of the given radiation.

Quality factor for x ray and gamma ray - One

Quality factor for Alpha - 20

Radiation Protection

General principles

Increasing the distance between radiation source and personnel:

a) Minimal handlers

b) Chemical restraint

c) Cassette holding device

d) Rotation of personnel

e) Use of shielding booth

f) Minimal fluoroscopy

Use of protective barriers- scattered radiation

a) **Aprons**: 0. 25mm lead lining-100Kv+lead rubber never fold the aprons

b) **Gloves and goggles**: 0. 33mm-100Kv,check for cracks.

c) **Location of x-ray plant**: corner of hospital, limited people movement, use of warning signs, wall 22cm thick concrete and lead lining with plywood.

Reduction of exposure factors and unnecessary radiography

Use of radiation monitoring devices

a) Film badge at waist level

b) Film badge at neck line

c) Thermo luminescent dosimeters (BARC, Trombay, Bombay)

d) Personal exposure meter

e) Pocket ionizing chamber

X-ray beam filters, collimators, tube lead shielding-aluminum filters: 2.5mm thickness

Persons below 18 years and pregnant women should be avoided.

Safety rules followed in radiograph

1. Should not allow person below 18 years and pregnant women in the room during exposure.
2. Personal rotation to minimize the exposure dose.
3. Avoid manual restraining or positioning
4. Use Protective devise
5. Never allow any part of body to primary x ray beam
6. Use collimeter to avoid primary beam
7. Use aluminum filter to remove soft x-rays
8. Use radiation monitoring devises.

□□□

28

Ultrasonography

Principles of ultrasonography and its applications in veterinary practice

Ultrasonography is an important modality for Tomography imaging of soft tissues. It is also used to quantitate the movement of structures and to access the patterns of blood flow. Ultrasound for medically diagnostic purposes was developed from SONAR (sound navigation and ranging) systems used to detect submarines. The human ear can detect frequencies in the range of 20-20000 Hz. Sound above this range is known as ultrasound which is inaudible. Most instruments used in diagnostic medicine use sound in the range of 1-10 MHz.

Principle-when any form of energy is applied to a quartz crystal it vibrates to produce waves. This wave strikes the various tissues and is reflected back to the quartz crystals, which in turn produces a corresponding electric current. This current is further processed by the machine, to be displayed as images. The image is displayed in various shades of grey depending on tissue density. e.g. bone appears white and fluid appears black. Selection of transducer depends on types of animals, organ and depth of organ. Sound waves travels in a pulse and when it is reflected back it become the echo. So it is pulse-echo principle used for ultra- sound imaging.

Production: Ultrasound is produced from Piezo electric crystal. When electric current is passed into the crystal, it undergoes deformation and emits sound waves of different frequency which are termed as ultrasound waves. This phenomenon is called Inverse Piezo electric effect. Depending on the size, shape and number of piezo electric crystal the frequency of the sound waves could be altered. Piezo electric crystals are housed in a transducer /Probe.

Properities of Ultra sound wave

- Frequency - is the number of times a wave is repeated per second. As the frequency increases, axial resolution increases, there will be more attenuation to the wave. The resistance exerted by the body tissue to the passage of sound is termed as **Acoustic impedence**.
- Like electromagnetic energy, ultrasound energy is transmitted through a medium or totally reflected back toward the point of generation or refracted (bent) or absorbed or attenuated (loose energy)
- In tissues, ultrasound is transmitted, absorbed, reflected or refracted
- $V= \lambda f$ V = velocity of sound λ = Waved length f = frequency
- Smaller the wave length, greater absorption of sound, greater resolution, lesser penetration.
- Sound transmitted by tissue by one molecular moving and transmitting energy to another.
- The penetration ability is controlled by the frequency of ultrasound wave. Shorter the frequency higher is the penetration.
- Velocity - The Velocity of ultrasound in tissues depends on tissue characteristics. In air containing organs (Lungs) propagation is maximum where as skeletal structures (Bones) propagation could be minimum and in parenchymatous organs (Liver) it is optimal.

Components of an ultrasonograph

1. Transducer

Function: To send and receive signals

Parts of transducer are Plastic housing, Acoustic insulator, Backing block, Electrodes, Piezo – electric crystal (Lead zerconate titanate).

Different types of transducer

1. Linear type: Thin rectangular clips lined side by side (60-256 crystal in line). Beam produced is rectangular (fig.109).
2. Convex type: Crystal arranged in curvilinear fashion, Image formed is of greater area (fig.110).
3. Sector type: Single crystal oscillates to provide fan shaped beam, Small size, more maneuverability. Used for thoracic and abdominal organs through small contact area (fig.111).

Small dog and cats → 7.5 to 10.0 MHz, Medium dogs→ 5MHz

Large dogs → 3.0 to 5.0 MHz, Large animals→ 2.0 to 3.5 MHz

2. Ultrasound beam

Beam has parallel sound waves. Three zones are found in beam- Fresnel, focal and Fraunhofer zones.

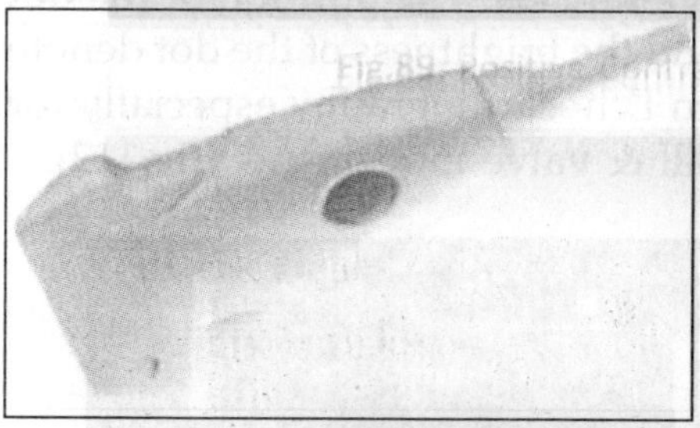

Fig.109. Linear Probe transducer

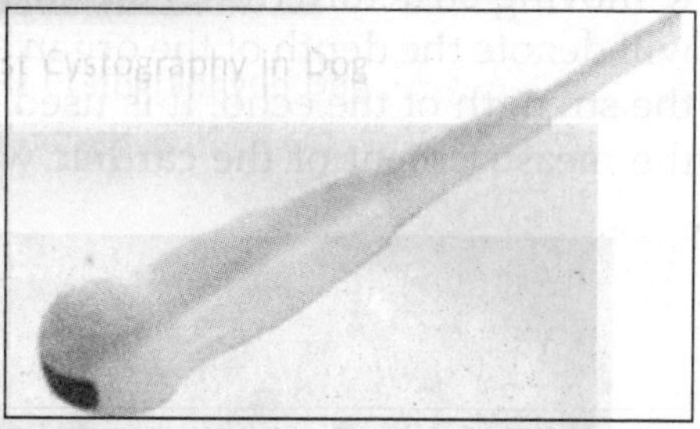

Fig.110. Convex Probe transducer

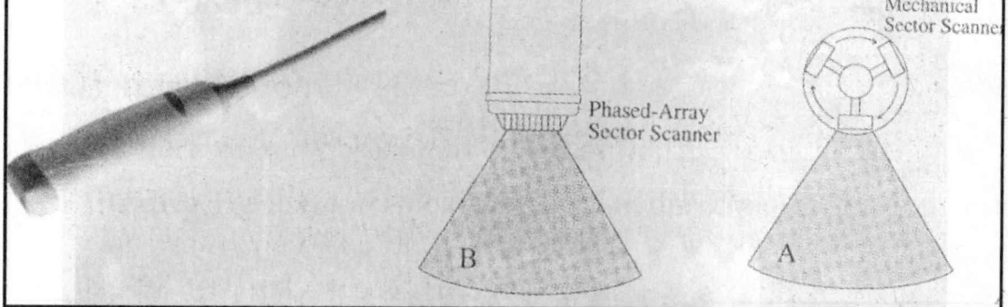

Fig.111. Sector Probe transducer

3. Display Modes

A-Mode (Amplitude mode): Supplies from, single wired Ultrasound beam is used, receiving echoes shown as peaks along horizontal line and height of each echo denotes the strength of echo. Height of peak is strength of echo, Horizontal axis is the depth of organ. Information about boundary of organ, anatomical relationship is obtained.

B-Mode (Brightness mode): Multiple Ultrasound beams are used. Returning echo is depicted as the dots and Brightness of the dot is directly proportional to the strength of the echo which is called as "Grey- Scale imaging". Image formed will be 2D image. most popular mode of display. Information regarding internal structure of organ can be obtained. Brightness denotes depth of organ. Commonly used for Echo cardiography.

TM- Mode (Time-Motion mode): Single Ultrasound beam is used. Returning echoes are depicted as dots (depth) along the vertical axis & moving structure (time) on horizontal axis. The position of the dot will denote the depth of the organ and the brightness of the dot denote the strength of the echo. It is used in Echocardiography especially for the measurement of the cardiac wall & valve movements (fig.112).

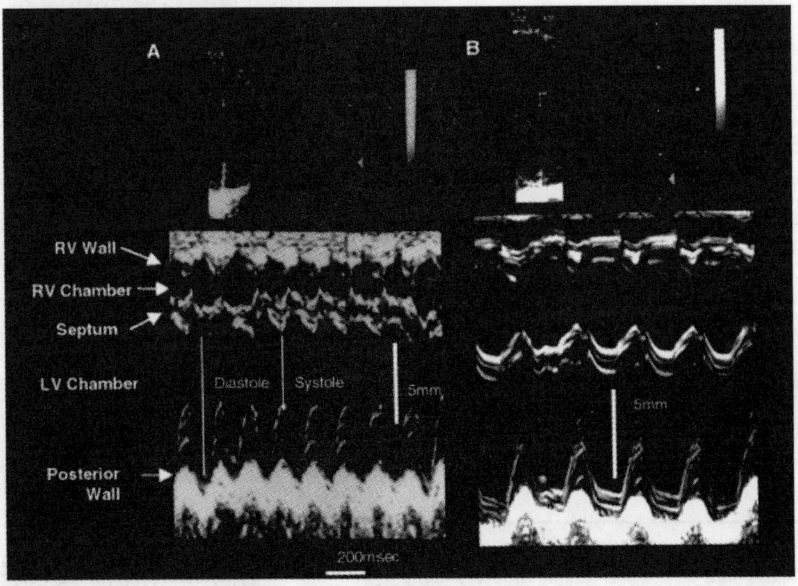

Fig.112. TM- Mode (Time-Motion mode) showing marked increase in RV and LV end diastolic chamber diameters

Real-Time Ultrasonography: The ability to see motion on the displayed ultrasound image. Real-time B-mode scanners display a moving gray scale image of cross sectional anatomy. Accomplished by sweeping a thin, focused Ultrasound beam across a triangular field of view in the patient any times/second. Saggital, transverse, dorsal or oblique planes through the body may be obtained by changing the transducer's orientation on the skin.

Preparation of the patient

Patient fasting, Administration of laxatives, antiflatuents, enema. Preparation of site by clipping/shaving and application of ultrasound gel.

Reflection and acoustic impedance: Echoes reflected from soft tissue interface towards the transducer form the basis of ultrasound image. The product of tissue density and sound velocity within the tissue is known as acoustic impedance. Bone and gas have very high and very low acoustic impedance respectively. Height of peak is strength of echo and Horizontal axis is the depth of organ.

Image interpretation

- **Hyper-echoic/echogenic/echo rich.** It is seen as bright images. E.g: bone or air.
- **Hypo- echoic/echo poor.** It is seen as grey image: moderate reflection. E.g:Liver
- **Anechoic/echo lucent/echo free black image**. fluid filled area. E.g: Urinary bladder

Interpretation based on Texture of organ

- Uniform/ regular homogenous
- Non-uniform/ irregular non homogenous
- Fine, coarse

Echo	Border	Possible diagnosis
Hyperechoie	Mostly irregular	Neoplasia, hematoma air bone
Hypoechoic	Smooth and distinct to irregular	Abscess, Lymphoma, neoplasia, hematoma
Anechoie	Smooth and distinct	Free peritoneal fluid, cyst, abscess, hematoma, fluid in GIT

Order of increasing echogenecity

Bile, urine
↓
Renal medulla
↓
Muscle
↓
Renal cortex
↓
Liver
↓
Storage fat
↓
Spleen
↓
Prostate
↓
Renal sinus
↓
Structural fat, vessel walls
↓
Bone, gas, organ boundries

When the ultrasound wave pass through tissue there will be three phenomenon :

1. Reflection
2. Refraction
3. Absorption

1. Ultrasound cannot penetrate skeletal structures

- 90-95% of Ultrasound wave which strikes bone is Reflected back it may not be useful for diagnostic purpose.
- Such structures of body reflecting most of Ultrasound are called HYPERECHOIC Structures

2. Muscle, tendon parenchymatous organs

- Ultrasound can able to penetrate these structures from 40-60% of which 30-40% gets reflected back.

- Such organs are called HYPOECHOIC.
- Most parenchymatous organs are HYPOECHOIC.

3. Hollow organs containing Liquid

- Like Urinary bladder, gallblader, Intestines.
- Here there is no resistance to Ultrasound penetration, then >95% beam passed through, neither absorbed nor reflected.
- Only 5% is reflected back carrying very minimal information of organ. Such organs are called ANECHOIC.

Selection of transducer

Depends on types of animal, organ & depth of organ.

Small dogs & cats	7.5-10 MHz
Medium dogs	5.0 MHz
Large dogs	3.0-5.0 MHz
Large animals	2.0-3.5 MHz
Dorsal liver of large dog	3.0 MHz
Spleen & left Kidney	5-7.5.0 MHz

Image storage

1. Polaroid camera: poor storage life, Fading of image when exposed to light.
2. Thermal printing: A printer attached to video monitor
3. Multiformat camera
4. Video cassette, VCD
5. Hard disk, floppy

Artifacts

Useless artifacts may be formed due to improper use of equipment, improper machine setting, improper scanning procedure and improper patient preparation.

Eg: Reverberation, Comet Tail, Mirror image, Side Lobe Effect, Slice Thickness Artifact and Refraction.

Useful artifacts: Enhance accurate interpretation, produced under proper technical condition. It is result of interaction between Ultrasound & matter.

E.g.: Acoustic Shadow and Acoustic Enhancement.

Reverberation: Produced as Largest source of positive artifact that is not real. Bouncing of echo between two interfaces.

a. External Reverberation - skin-transducer interface (fig.113).

   External reverberation artifact (solid arrows) created by air interposition between transducer and the animal (small arrow heads). Small internal reverberation artifact is associated with air filled bowel (open arrow.

b. Internal Reverberation - internal reflector such as bone or air (fig.114).

   Internal reverberation artifact created by a superficially located air-filled bowel. Note the repetation of equally parallel lines. Second image shows Schematic representation of the mechanism of reverberation. Numerous linear reverberation artifacts are created by the gas in the bowel. The sound is entirely reflected from gas and bounces back and forth between the probe and the gas, creating multiple repeating echoes, each becoming weaker and occurring at the greater depth with one ultrasound pulse.

Comet tail: Caused by highly reflective interface as between air and fluid such as in the partially consolidated lungs or metal objects. Interface between bowel wall & bowel gas (fig.115).

Mirror image: Occurs at highly reflective interface. Returning echo reach the transducer under a time delay and seen as a highly echogenecity interface (fig.116 mirror image artifact of liver and gall bladder. The shape of the diaphragm causes some of the returning echos to be delayed).

Eg. Diaphragm - lung interface, here liver look as if displaced into thoracic cavity

Side lobe effect - Lateral displacement of structure not aligned with sound beam. Organ is seen as laterally displaced, though organ is present in normal position. Occurs in diaphragm, bladder, gall bladder and with air.

Slice thickness artifact: In the bladder & gall bladder a variant of slide lobe artifact is slice thickness artifact which mimics the presence of sediment in the bladder/gall bladder.

- True sediment –flat surface.
- Pseudo sediment - curved surface

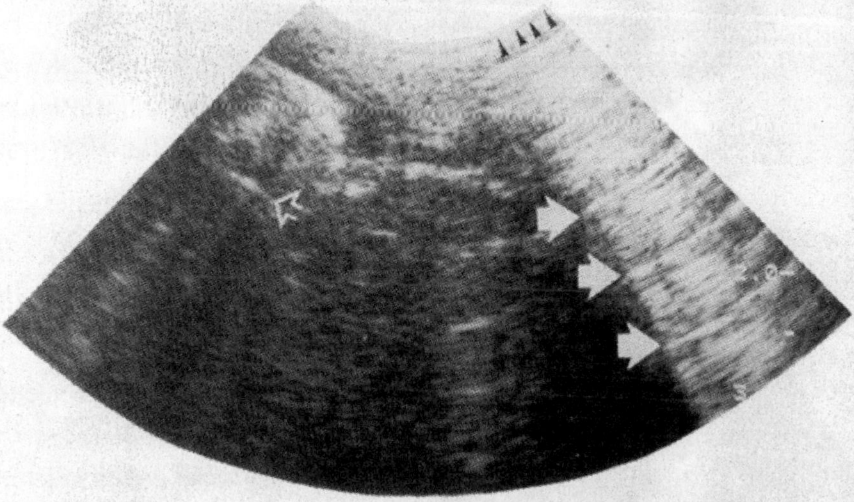

Fig.113. External Reverberation Artifact created by air interposition between the trasducer and the animal

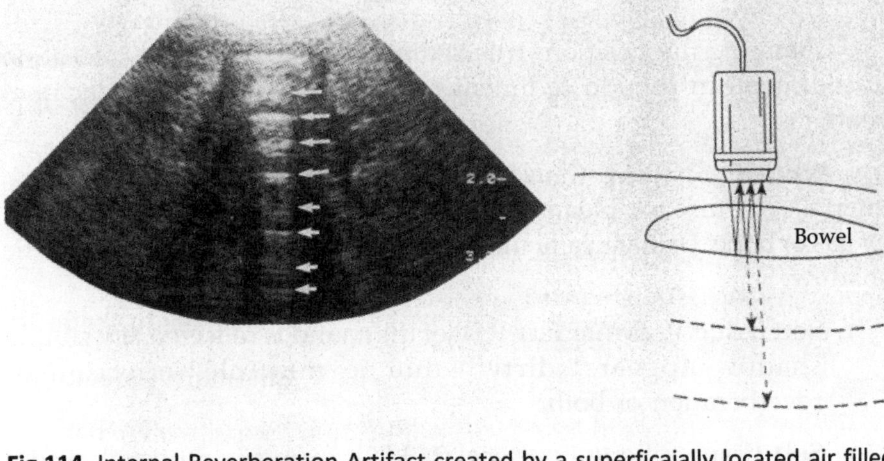

Fig.114. Internal Reverberation Artifact created by a superficaially located air filled bowel.

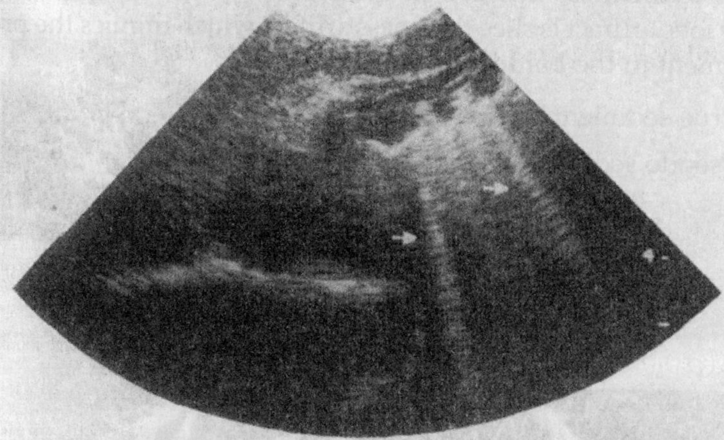

Fig.115. Comet Tail Artifact

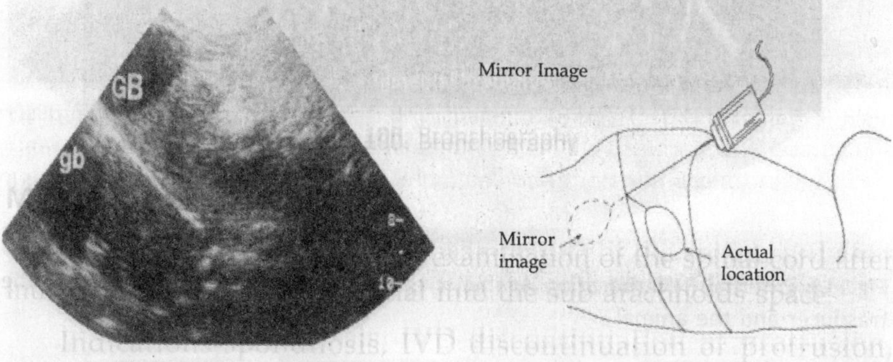

Fig.116. Mirror Image (GB-actual image and gb- mirror image)

Changing the position- true sediment interface changes location of sediment, in pseudo sediment remain perpendicular to incident beam

Acousitc Shadow: Caused by Reflection of sound at an acoustic interface. - Pulse unable to reach the deeper structures. It is produced by gas or bone. Urinary calliculi and gall stones- produce clean acoustic shadow.

- Soft tissue – gas interface 99% of the sound is reflected & resulting shadow appears 'dirty' –due to multiple reflection or reverberation or both.
- Soft tissue – bone interface, 2/3rd of sound is reflected and a significant portion is absorbed.

- Complete absence of reverberation & 'clean' shadow
- Barium in a segment of bowel – produce clean shadow – attenuation due to reflection.

Edge Shadowing: Seen distal to the lateral margins of cystic structures. Seen in bladder, gall bladder, kidney.

Enhancement: Opposite to attenuation shadowing. Echoes from deeper tissues are amplified and appear as area of increased brightness. Seen distal to the gall bladder and urinary bladder. Helps in differentiating cystic structure from solid and hypoechoic masses.

Uses of Ultrasound

1. Obstetric or pregnancy: Presence or absence of a pregnancy – This is done by noting the presence of a Gestational Sac i.e. the sac that contains the fetus. The scan also helps identify the location of the pregnancy – whether intrauterine or extra uterine. The latter is referred to as an ectopic pregnancy.
2. Assess the growth and development of the fetus.
3. Assess the amount of fluid surrounding the fetus i.e. liquor amnii.
4. To detect abnormality in visceral organs (inflammation, tumor, cyst, effusions etc.)
5. Placental localization and assess the amount of fluid surrounding the fetus i.e. liquor amnii.
6. Lithotripsy and Ultrasound therapy
7. Discriminating nature of tissue
8. Ocular examination and Cardiac evaluation
9. Biopsy of organ/tissue
10. Diagnosis of myopathis
11. Ultrasound therapy
12. Ocular examination
13. Cardiac evaluation
14. Biopsy of organ/tissue
15. Aspiration of content to know whether it is normal/abnormal
16. Diagnosis of lesions in fluid filled cavities

Diagnostic applications of ultrasound

Site	Application for
1. Abdomen	Pressence of fluid, peritonitis, lipoma, hernia
2. Liver	Cyst, hematomas, necrosis, neoplasm
3. Gall bladder	Obstruction, calculi
4. Kidney	Size, cyst, calculi, blood, clot, abnormalities of renal pelvis, ureter
5. Bladder	Calculi, blood, clot, neoplasm
6. Male genital system	Testicles for size, neoplasm, atrophy, prostatitis, benign prostate hyperplasia
7. Female genital system	Status of follicle, ovary size, cystic ovary, size of uterus, pregnancy, pyometra, neoplasm
8. Salivary gland	Cyst, sialolith
9. Eye	Intraocular neoplasm, blood clot, cataract, lens dislocation
10. Musculoskeletal system	Muscle, ligament, tendon tear, joint disease, effusion

Advantages of ultrasound

- It is a non- invasive diagnostic technique
- No preparation of patient
- Helps in visualization of anomaly
- Technique can be performed on any patient i.e., old, dyspnoeic and comatose patients
- Useful in differentiation of soft tissue abnormalities
- Very minimal risk of producing harmful effects
- Biopsy can be taken for accurate diagnosis

Disadvantages

- Clipping of hairs and cleaning of the skin which is of aesthetic importance
- Application of coupling medium such as mineral oil, aqueous gel - desquamation of cells leading to metastasis.

Adverse effects associated with ultrasound

- Potassium leakage from red blood cells
- Platelet aggregation
- Damage to tissue endothelium.

Contraindications

- Thrombophlebitis or other blood clot conditions
- Fractures
- Epiphyseal injuries
- Vascular diseases (embolus formation - plaque rupture)
- Spinal column injuries (treat low back pain with caution)
- Cancer (danger of metastases)
- Do not apply directly over heart (pacemaker concerns).

□□□

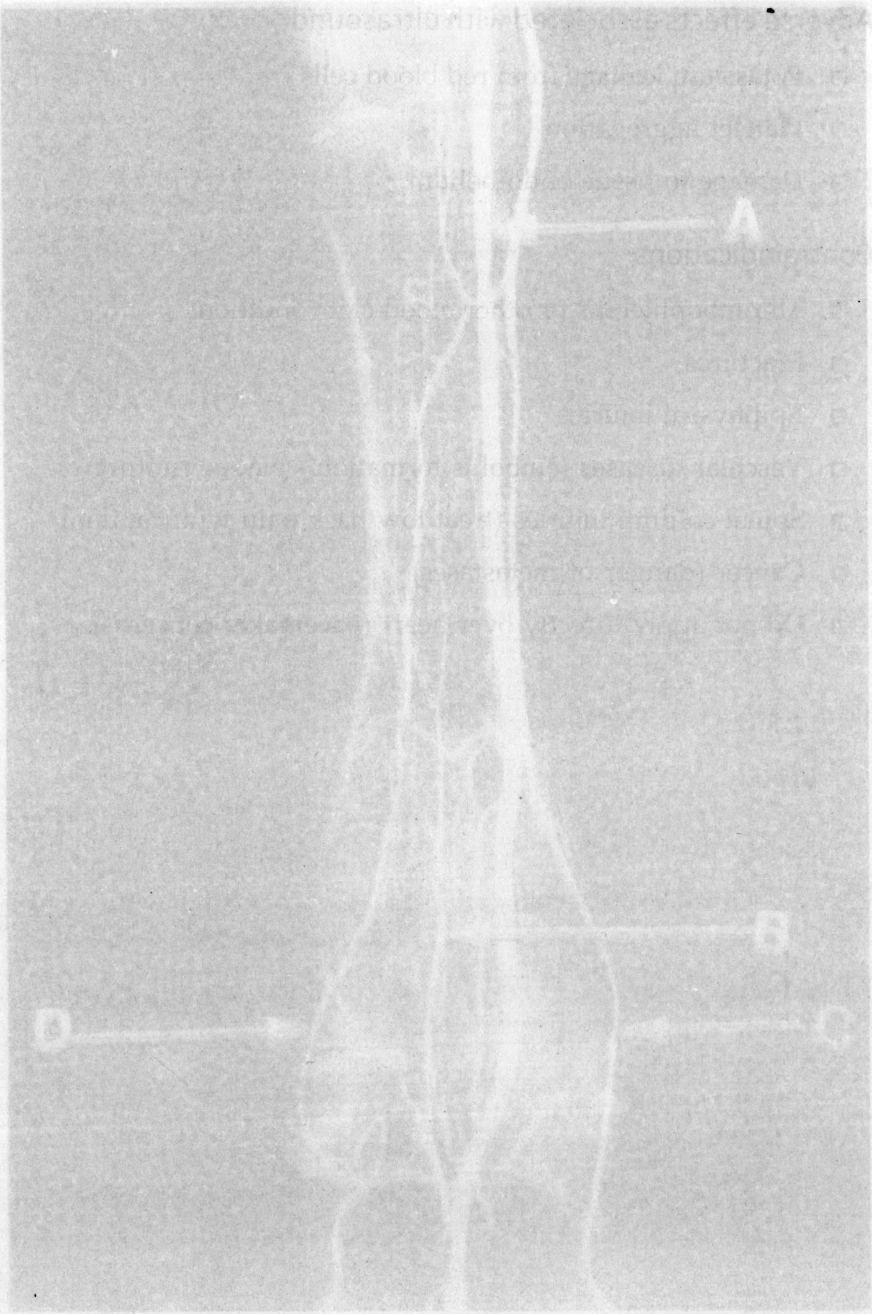

Fig.103. Arteriography (Metacarpal region in buffalo calf). A. Great metacarpal artery; B. Dorsal metacarpal artery; C.Medial palmar metacarpal artery; D. lateralpalmar metacarpal artery

29

Principles of Radiation Therapy

Dr R. Eberlin (1906-1912) was the first person to report radiation therapy in veterinary practice. The basic of radio therapy is to kill the tumour cells by ionizing radiation. Treatment of cancer involves Surgery, Chemotherapy, Radiation Therapy, Recombinant DNA technology and Radiation Therapy can be combined with the other methods of treatment.

Radiation therapy includes

1. **Radiosensitivity** - Refers to susceptibility of cells or tissues to a given dose of absorbed radiation. Dose required is variable according to the type of cells.
2. **Radiocurability** - Complete regression of tumour and survival of patient for a minimum of two years after the treatment.
3. **Radio Response** - Degree to which either normal or neoplastic tissue will undergo visible change both during and after the therapy.
4. **Radio Isotopes** - Radionuclide having same atomic number with difference in atomic weight. They are implanted in or on the affected part. Eg. Cobalt, Cesium.

C_6^{14} Superscript-Mass number

Subscript-Atomic number

Isotopes of some heavy elements such as cobalt, cesiums etc are unstable and active. These unstable nuclides undergo process of spontaneous decay to form stable nuclides by process of radioactive decay. During the process of this decay, there is emission of radiation energy from the isotopes. Such isotopes are called Radioisotopes or radionuclide. Such Isotopes whenever implanted in cancerous tissues they release radiant energy and capable of destroying cell which helps in regression of tumour.

Nuclear medicine - Branch of medical science employ the radioisotope both for diagnosis and treatment of various diseases

Scintigraphy - Diagnostic technique where isotopes used for early diagnosis of skeletal and parenchymatous organ disorders.

Properties of Radionuclide

- Emit gamma radiation
- Non toxic
- Suitable physical T 1/2
- Short biological T 1/2
- Capable of labeling pharmaceutical compound

Mechanism of action

- Target theory or direct theory – Radiation directly acts on DNA molecule or linkage where it can produce damage or death of cells
- Indirect theory- Radiation acts on cell leading to production of hot radicals peroxidase) which lead to cell death.

Tissue tolerance to radiotherapy

Neoplasm lethal dose - Normal tissue tolerance dose

Eg-200 rads for lens

2000 rads for kidneys

4000 rads for brain

Therapeutic ratio - Ratio of normal tissue tolerance to neoplasm's lethal dose.

Indication for radiation therapy

- Localized solid neoplasm's
- When surgery fails.
- Tumor without metastasis
- For debulking-Then subsequent surgery

Methods of radiotherapy

- Reoxygenation
- Repopulation
- Redistribution
- Repair

Radionuclide used

- Brain – Pertechnetate M99 technitium
- Liver – Technitium sulphor collide
- Kidney- Technitium Chelate
- Skeleton- Technitium M99 Pyrophasphate
- Placenta- Technitium labelled human serum albumin
- Lungs – Technitium labelled micro sphere

Techniques of radiation therapy

1. **Teletherapy**: Source of radiation is kept at a distance from the lesion
   - Superficial X-ray therapy (60-100 kV)
   - Deep X-ray therapy (200-300Kv)
   - Super voltage therapy (1-20mv)
   - Particulate beam therapy (proton, electron and neutron beams are used)
2. **Brachytherapy:** Source of radiation will be on the surface or within the parenchyma of tumour Radionuclides used in the form of needles, seeds or grains which are implanted on the tumour.

A. Interstitial Brachytherapy : Source of radiation kept with in the parenchyma of lesion.

Advantage

- Release of continuous low radiation with in the tumour
- High total dose can be achieved
- Implantation is easier
- Duration of treatment is shorter

Disadvantage

Implantation is invasive and requires special training

B. Pleiso therapy : Also called as surface Brachytherapy, Source of radiation kept on the surface

C. Systemic Brachytherapy: Radioisotope are administered intravascularly so that its acts on specific tumour. Eg. Leukemia and thyroid tumour.

Choice of Treatment

1. Small superficial skin lesion- superficial radiation therapy
2. Deep lesions of skin – super voltage or deep therapy
3. Shallow or deep moderate size organ- super voltage or particulate beam therapy.

Leukemia or thyroid cancer

Complication

1. Immediate: Hair loss, moist eczema, bone marrow depression.
2. Latent- Onset of leukemia, onset of new cancer, production of lethal genes, shortening of life span of patient.
3. Complications depends on the area affected
   - Ophthalmic neoplasm's irradiation: Conjunctival keratitis/ cataract etc.
   - Bone: Fracture/Sepsis/Osteochondrosis/sarcoma

Measurement of radiation hazards and their prevention by adaptation of safety measures Units of measurement, electron volt (eV) it is a unit of x- ray energy as 1000 eV and million eV.

ROENTGEN is unit of exposure to x ray measures quantity of ionization.

- Radiation absorbed dose (rad) unit of absorbed following exposure to ionization
- Roentgen equelent man (rem)=rad× quality factors.
- Grey(Gy) one joule of energy per kg of absorbed material.

Factors Affecting Radiation Hazards

1. Dose of radiation
2. Duration of exposure
3. Type of body tissues
4. Species of animals

Applications

1. Localized solid cancers
2. Recurrence of tumor inspite of surgery
3. Primary tumors with metastasis
4. Detect functional disorders of kidney, liver and G.I. tract

Limitations

- High cost
- Safety measures
- Etiological non specificity
- Difficulty in interpretation specially in skeletal system

Labelling of Isotope

Radioisotopic labelling

Radioisotopic labelling is a technique for tracking the passage of a sample of substance through a system. The substance is "labelled" by including radionuclides in its chemical composition. When these decay, their presence can be determined by detecting the radiation they emit. Radioisotopic labelling is a special case of **isotopic labelling**. For these purposes, a particularly useful type of radioactive decay is positron emission. When a positron collides with an electron, it releases two high-energy photons travelling in diametrically opposite directions. If the positron is produced within a solid object, it is likely to do this before travelling more than a millimetre. If both of these photons can be detected, the location of the decay event can be determined very precisely.

Different kinds of labelling

Most frequently, proteins are labelled with ^{15}N and ^{13}C. ^{2}H labelling is used for proteins of larger molecular weight.

Sources of isotopes used for labelling

The simplest labelling, and also the cheapest one is ^{15}N, because ^{15}N ammonia is quite cheap. ^{13}C is more expensive, because it requires the synthesis (most commonly - biosynthesis) of ^{13}C glucose, some expression systems allow use of cheaper $^{13}CO_2$.

Radioimmunoconjugates

Conjugation of radionuclides to antibodies can be used for two purposes: therapy and imaging. In the case of therapy a radionuclide with a short pathlength (beta emitters) is used so that the damage is limited to the targeted area. For imaging, radionuclides with long pathlengths are used (gama emitters), which can be detected by an appropriate camera.

One feature of radioimmunoconjugates is that, even if the antibody is targeted specifically to a cell bearing the appropriate antigen, the killing mechanism spreads from that targeted cell. This can lead to unwanted toxicity to normal tissues. However, it can be an advantage because the radiation may kill cells that need to be killed, but are not targeted by the antibody. This might include the blood vessels feeding a tumor or tumor cells that the antibody cannot reach.

E-selectin is an adhesion molecule that is expressed only on activated endothelium, seen at sites of inflammation. It is a highly specific marker of inflammation, but being expressed on the luminal surface of endothelium it is highly accessible to antibodies in the vasculature. Antibodies to E-Selection have been used to image rheumatoid arthritis and inflammatory bowel disease, as well as to locate occult infection in patient with acquired immunodeficiency syndrome.

Most imaging is done with gama emitting antibodies, which can be detected with a gamma camera, using standard nuclear medicine facilities such as single photon emission computed tomography (SPECT). However, there are alternatives, including the delivery of positron emitters for positron emission tomography (PET) and magnetic contrast agents for magnetic resonance imaging (MRI). Antibodies have even been conjugated onto bubbles, with a view of developing targetable contrast agents for ultrasonography. Each imaging modality has particular advantages, giving complementary information for clinical diagnosis.

Biological use of Isotopes

1. Isotopes

Isotopes for a given atomic element are a variety of atoms with the same number of protons, but a different number of neutrons. Isotopes occurring naturally in an organism or injected can be used for imaging internal structure and function. These are highly radioactive, short-lived radioisotopes. Longer-lived radioisotopes are useful for placing organisms in the geological record, aiding determination of evolutionary rates.

2. Nuclear Magnetic Resonance Imaging (NMRI)

NMRI is a visualization technique used to image the internal bodily structures and functions. Isotopes naturally occurring in the body that have a magnetic moment will process around an axis along the direction of a strong external magnetic field. Hydrogen isotopes in water molecules throughout the body are commonly used.

Protons with a magnetic moment enter a state of excitation when the magnets of the NMRI scanner are on. When the magnetic fields are turned off, the protons release their excitation energy at resonance radio frequencies that are detected by the NMRI scanner. Difference in tissues is measurable because the protons in different tissues return to their equilibrium state at different rates.

3. Diagnostic Radiopharmaceuticals

Every organ in our bodies acts differently from a chemical point of view. Doctors and chemists have identified a number of chemicals which are absorbed by specific organs. The thyroid, for example, takes up iodine, the brain consumes quantities of glucose and so on. With this knowledge, radiopharmacists are able to attach various radioisotopes to biologically active substances. Once a radioactive form of one of these substances enters the body, it is incorporated into the normal biological processes and excreted in the usual ways.

Diagnostic radiopharmaceuticals can be used to examine blood flow to the brain, functioning of the liver, lungs, heart or kidneys, to assess bone growth, and to confirm other diagnostic procedures. Another important use is to predict the effects of surgery and assess changes since treatment.

The amount of the radiopharmaceutical given to a patient is just sufficient to obtain the required information before its decay. The radiation dose received is medically insignificant. The patient experiences no discomfort during the test and after a short time there is no trace that the test was ever done. The non-invasive nature of this technology, together with the ability to observe an organ functioning from outside the body, makes this technique a powerful diagnostic tool.

A radioisotope used for diagnosis must emit gamma rays of sufficient energy to escape from the body and it must have a half-life short enough for it to decay away soon after imaging is completed.

The radioisotope most widely used in medicine is technetium-99m, employed in some 80% of all nuclear medicine procedures. It is an isotope of the artificially-produced element technetium and it has almost ideal characteristics for a nuclear medicine scan. These are:

- It has a half-life of six hours which is long enough to examine metabolic processes yet short enough to minimise the radiation dose to the patient.
- Technetium-99m decays by a process called "isomeric"; which emits gamma rays and low energy electrons. Since there is no high energy beta emission the radiation dose to the patient is low.

- The low energy gamma rays it emits easily escape the human body and are accurately detected by a gamma camera. Once again the radiation dose to the patient is minimised.
- The chemistry of technetium is so versatile it can form tracers by being incorporated into a range of biologically-active substances to ensure that it concentrates in the tissue or organ of interest.

Its logistics also favour its use. Technetium generators, a lead pot enclosing a glass tube containing the radioisotope, are supplied to hospitals from the nuclear reactor where the isotopes are made. They contain molybdenum-99, with a half-life of 66 hours, which progressively decays to technetium-99. The Tc-99 is washed out of the lead pot by saline solution when it is required. After two weeks or less the generator is returned for recharging.

A similar generator system is used to produce rubidium-82 for PET imaging from strontium-82 - which has a half-life of 25 days.

Myocardial Perfusion Imaging (MPI) uses thallium-201 chloride or technetium-99m and is important for detection and prognosis of coronary artery disease.

For PET imaging, the main radiopharmaceutical is Fluoro-deoxy glucose (FDG) incorporating F-18 - with a half-life of just under two hours, as a tracer. The FDG is readily incorporated into the cell without being broken down, and is a good indicator of cell metabolism.

In diagnostic medicine, there is a strong trend for using more cyclotron-produced isotopes such as F-18 as PET and CT/PET become more widely available. However, the procedure needs to be undertaken within two hours reach of a cyclotron.

4. Therapeutic Radiopharmaceuticals

For some medical conditions, it is useful to destroy or weaken malfunctioning cells using radiation. The radioisotope that generates the radiation can be localised in the required organ in the same way it is used for diagnosis - through a radioactive element following its usual biological path, or through the element being attached to a suitable biological compound. In most cases, it is beta radiation which causes the destruction of the damaged cells. This is radionuclide therapy (RNT) or radiotherapy. Short-range radiotherapy is known as **brachytherapy,** and this is becoming the main means of treatment.

Although radiotherapy is less common than diagnostic use of radioactive material in medicine, it is nevertheless widespread, important and growing. An ideal therapeutic radioisotope is a strong beta emitter with just enough gamma to enable imaging, eg lutetium-177. This is prepared from ytterbium-176 which is irradiated to become Yb-177 which decays rapidly to Lu-177. Yttrium-90 is used for treatment of cancer, particularly non-Hodgkin's lymphoma, and its more widespread use is envisaged, including for arthritis treatment. Lu-177 and Y-90 are becoming the main RNT agents.

Iodine-131 and phosphorus-32 are also used for therapy. Iodine-131 is used to treat the thyroid for cancers and other abnormal conditions such as hyperthyroidism (over-active thyroid). In a disease called Polycythemia vera, an excess of red blood cells is produced in the bone marrow. Phosphorus-32 is used to control this excess.

A new and still experimental procedure uses boron-10, which concentrates in the tumour. The patient is then irradiated with neutrons which are strongly absorbed by the boron, to produce high-energy alpha particles which kill the cancer.

For targeted alpha therapy (TAT), actinium-225 is readily available, from which the daughter bismuth-213 can be obtained (via 3 alpha decays) to label targeting molecules. The bismuth is obtained by elution from an Ac-225/Bi-213 generator similar to the Mo-99/Tc-99 one. Bi-213 has a 46-minute half-life. The actinium-225 (half-life 10 days) is formed from radioactive decay of radium-225, the decay product of long-lived thorium-229, which is obtained from decay of uranium-233, which is formed from Th-232 by neutron capture in a nuclear reactor.

Considerable medical research is being conducted worldwide into the use of radionuclides attached to highly specific biological chemicals such as immunoglobulin molecules (monoclonal antibodies). The eventual tagging of these cells with a therapeutic dose of radiation may lead to the regression or even cure of some diseases.

□□□

30

Principles and Application of Computed Tomography

Computed Tomography (CT): Computed tomography is a diagnostic modality that is fundamentally different X- ray method in which an organ is scanned in successive layers by narrow beams of X rays in such a way that the transmission of X ray photons across a particular layer can be measured by means of a computer and used to construct a picture of that organ (fig.117).

OR

It can also be defined as digital imaging technique that uses x-ray energy and computer processing to make cross-sectional (transverse) images of structures.

Tomography is a Greek word **Tomos** – Slice **Graphein** – to write CT number is calibrated in Hounsfield unit (Hu) with water as reference of Zero Hu.

Principle

The patient is scanned by narrow beams of X rays. X ray tube Collimator and Detectors are fixed to a common frame. The rays passed are detected by collimator sensing device. Both X rays source and Detectors scan across the patient parts in 160 different planes and this is repeated for 360º. Then about 360 X 160 readings is taken by Detector. Data is stored & picture is reconstructed with the data. Image of a cross section can be formed by projecting many beams at many angles into the edge of the desired slice. The more fine the rays, more fine the details will be seen.

How it Works

X-ray tube
(detectors, collimator)
↓
Tissue
↓
Sensing device
↓
Computer
↓
Image

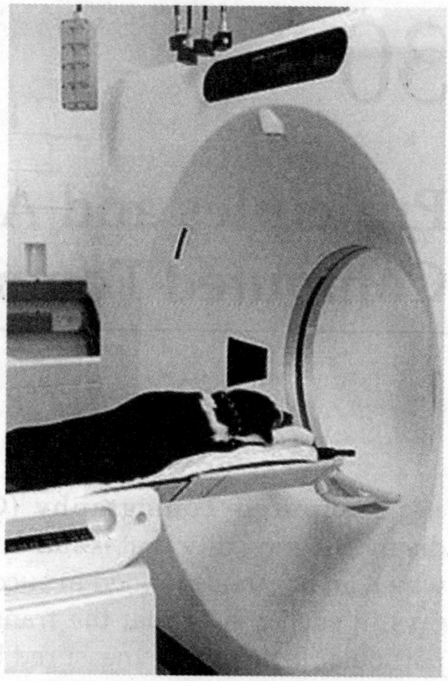

Fig.117. Small Animal Hospital CT Scan

Parts: It is a circular ring like machine with a large hole in the centre (like a dough nut) and a movable table.

- Gantry
- Table
- The x-ray tube
- Collimator, detectors
- Sensors
- CT computer

Components

- Unit for data acquisition – operating console, a patient handling table & a Gantry (portion which houses X ray source, collimator and detectors)
- Unit for image display & manipulation – Image display console
- Unit for data analysis – computer.

Types of CT

1. Third generation CT
2. Fourth generation CT
3. Axial tomography – designed to acquire a single slice at a time

4. Multislice CT – here more than one detector rings are used in CT Angiography
5. Helical or Spiral CT – as Gantry rotates the table also is in continuous motion
6. DRR CT – posses dual X ray tubes used in cardiac imaging
7. Electron beam CT – ideal for coronary arterial studies & cardiac Imaging.

Preparation: The animal should be well hydrated before procedure. Any metal objects should be removed. Animal should be anaesthetized to avoid movements. Contrast medium injections are given just before scanning. Food should be given 4 to 6 hours before scanning. Animal should be supported with pillows. Animal should be immobilized using tapes.

Position

- Head - Sternal recumbency
- Cervical spine - Sternal recumbency
- Thoracic, lumbar, and lumbosacral regions - Dorsal recumbency

Parts to be Scanned

- Brain, blood vessel, eye, inner ear, sinuses
- Neck, shoulder, cervical spine, Lumbar spine
- Chest, heart, aorta, lung, mediastinum, thorax
- Upper abdomen, liver, kidney, spleen, pancreas, G.I.tract
- Hand, feet, ankles, leg, arm, jaws.

PROCESS OF CT

X-ray source rotate around the object

↓

Data scan taken progresively

↓

Combining the data by Tomograph reconstruction procedure

↓

Data are arranged in a matrix in memory

↓

Reconstruction of each volume elements

↓

Through back projection reverse the acquisition geometry & store it in another memory

↓

Data can be displayed or photographed

↓

Further processing like multiplanar reconstruction is applied

Clinical Applications

1. Intracranial neoplasia, non neoplastic brain disease, or middle/ inner disease

   More sensitive than MRI for acute hemorrhage, soft tissue calcification, and intracranial mass.

   Less sensitive than MRI for edema, infarcts, low grade masses, and caudal fossa masses.

2. Hydrocephalus: Generalized or localized ventricular enlargement

3. Haemorrhage:

   Acute hemorrhage (24-72 hrs) - increased opacity

   Chronic (>72 hrs) - decreased opacity

   Edema-patchy areas of decreased opacity that are non-enhancing

4. Meningiomas and Gliomas

5. Choroid plexus papilloma

6. Pituitary macro adenoma: Mid-ventral fossa of the cranial vault, displace the 3rd ventricle dorsally, Enhance uniformly, and may exhibit a "*mushroom cloud*" shape. Post-contrast, transverse CT image with pituitary macroadenoma. a markedly-enhancing, sharply-marginated mass that is centered over the pituitary fossa can be noticed.

7. Otitis media: Increased soft tissue opacity in the bulla lumen. If Chronic, then thickening and sclerosis of the bulla walls or expansion of the bulla are noticed. Focal mineral opacities or otoliths may also be visible.

8. Spine: Intervertebral disc disease, spinal stenosis, or spinal masses.

- Less sensitive-discriminating soft tissues within the spinal canal.
- More sensitive-soft tissue calcifications, cortical bone spurs, degenerative changes in the articular process joints.

9. Intervertebral disc: **Type I** disc herniation: visible as either single or multiple bone opacity masses in the intervertebral canal, intervertebral foramina, or extraforaminal region.

   Type II disc herniation: Circumferential bulging of the annulus, narrowing of the intervertebral disc spaces, Endplate sclerosis, and endplate bone spurs (spondylosis deformans).

Advantages of CT over radiography

1. It is non invasive & painless method
2. Eliminates the superimposition of the underlying structures
3. Multiplanar reformatted imaging is possible
4. High contrast resolution so that hard & soft tissue are easily visible
5. CT – used for examining blood vessels of brain, kidney, lungs & also for screening arterial diseases
6. Displays the image digitally so normal & abnormal areas detected easily
7. Detects more subtle tissue density differences than radiography
8. Operators can adjust the contrast (window width) and brightness (window level)
9. Offers detailed views of many types of tissue
10. CT examinations are fast and simple
11. To guide radiotherapy, needle biopsies, and other minimally invasive procedures
12. CT can eliminate the need for invasive exploratory surgery and surgical biopsy
13. For a wide range of clinical problems.

Limitations of CT

1. Exposure to X rays similar to radiography or even more
2. Risk of serious allergic reaction to iodine-containing contrast

3. Soft tissues may be obscured by nearby bone structures
4. Very fine soft-tissue details –MRI is preferred.
5. Risk in pregnant animals
6. Patients with kidney diseases should not undergo contrast CT
7. Blocked blood vessels make the interpretation of CT difficult.

Artifacts

1. **Streaks:** Dark lines radiating from corners, It may be due to insufficient X ray tube current or Insufficient penetration of X ray
2. **Ray artifacts:** Images of one or many rings appear within the image. This is the fault of detector
3. **Noise artifacts:** Appear as grains on the image due to thin slice thickness
4. **Motion artifacts:** Caused by movements of object
5. **Wind mill artifacts:** Streaking appearance, Corrected by filtration
6. **Beam hardening artifacts:** Cupped appearance.

□□□

31

Magnetic Resonance and Imaging (MRI)

It is a non invasive technique, highly sensitive, accurate and detailed image, along with good contrast, spatial resolution and multiplanar capability without radiation hazards (fig.118).

Principle

Radio waves

↓

Proton Nuclei of hydrogen atom)

↓

Magnetic field

↓

Excited and then relaxed

↓

Radio signals

↓

Scanner

↓

Computer processed to form image

Properties

1. Magnetic force used is 1-2 tesla, about 30,000 times stronger than earth magnetic field.
2. Body protons are most abundant in hydrogen atoms of water. So MRI image shows differences in water content in different tissues.
3. Grey and white matter in the brain can be distinguished.

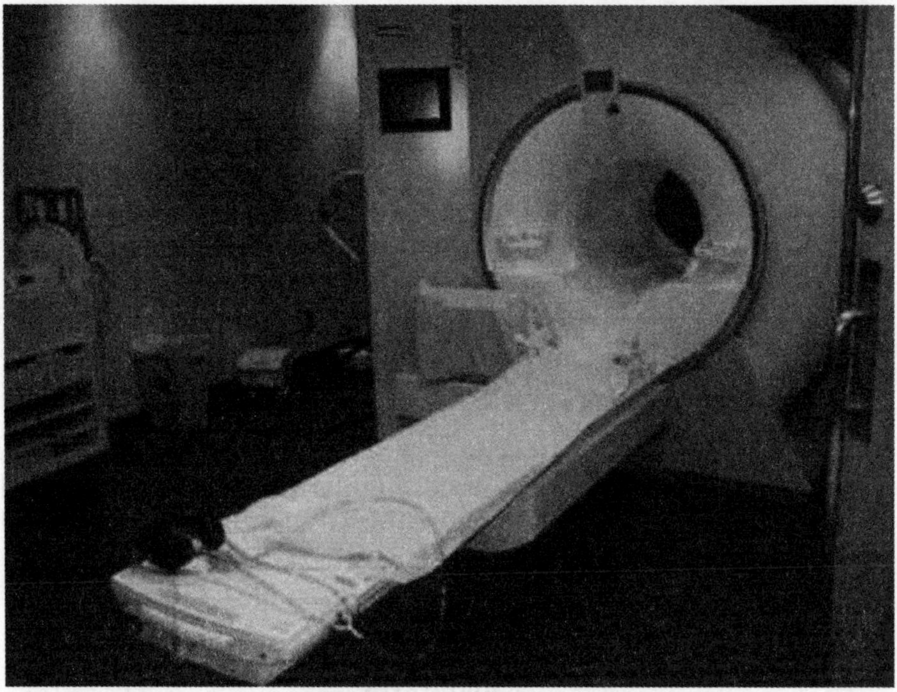

Fig.118 – Magnetic Resonance and Imaging

Application

- Useful in detection of conditions like seizures, chronic cervical pain, upper and lower motor neuron diseases, lumbosacral instability,
- Stroke or thromboembolism, Pituitary based tumor.
- To diagnose neurological, musculoskeletal, CVS disorders, herniated disc, arthritis,
- Small tears, injuries to ligaments, tendons, muscles can be diagnosed at early stage
- MRI cardiac - detailed blood vessels without contrast material (non i_2 agents gadolinium) supermagnetic contrast agent iron oxide nanoparticles
- Ophthalmology - blindness, pupil size changes, bulging eye can be diagnosed.
- Internal Medicine - liver, kidney, spleen, adrenal problems

- Head and nasal neoplasia or soft tissue neoplasia
- Other - sneezing, gagging, head shaking or flinching, or based on your primary care veterinarian recommendations
- After heart attack-to see whether blood flow is blocked in chambers of heart damage to heart muscles
- MRI have created movie like changes beating heart to diagnose CVS disease
- MRI angiography atherosclerosis, arterial aneurysm.

Precautions

- MRI uses strong magnetic field so can pull any ferromagnetic metal objects–prosthetic hip, IUD, artifical heart valve (heart pacemaker)
- Surgical plates, pins, staples and screws pose no risk during MRI, if more than 4-6 weeks
- Dyes tattoos, permanent eye liner contain metallic iron oxide could heat up during MRI
- Magnetic field will not effect tooth filling, but distort images at facial area or brain
- Hair pins, jewellary hearing aids, eyeglasses and any dental work should be avoided.
- Pregnant animals should be avoided
- Animals should be sedated close confinement or claustrophobic.

How procedure performed

- Patient comfortably positioned on special table that slides into MRI systems
- Depending on how many images taken generally takes 15-45 minutes
- Contrast materials used enhance visibility of tissues or blood vessels
- MRI takes 2-6 imaging sequences, each sequence own degree contrast and shows cross section in several planes right to left, front to back, upper to lower.

Advantages

1. Images of the soft-tissue structures of the body such as the heart, lungs, liver and other organs are clearer and more detailed than with other imaging methods.
2. MRI can help physicians evaluate the function as well as the structure of many organs.
3. The detail makes MRI an invaluable tool in early diagnosis and evaluation of tumors.
4. MRI contrast material is less likely to produce an allergic reaction than the iodine-based materials used for conventional X-rays and CT scanning.
5. MRI enables the detection of abnormalities that might be obscured by bone with other imaging methods.
6. MRI provides a fast, non-invasive alternative to x-ray, angiography for diagnosing problems of the heart and cardiovascular system.
7. Exposure to radiation is avoided.
8. Detailed images of blood vessels and blood flow are obtained without having to insert a catheter directly into the area of interest, so that there is no risk of damaging an artery or in the case of the brain, causing a stroke.
9. The procedure itself is shorter than after a traditional catheter angiogram. As well, there is no recovery time with the procedure, unlike the 4 to 6 hours needed for catheter angiography.
10. MRI is less costly than catheter angiography.

Risks

1. An undetected metal implant may be affected by the strong magnetic field.
2. MRI is generally avoided in the first 12 weeks of pregnancy.
3. Doctors usually use other methods of imaging such as ultrasound on pregnant women, unless there is a strong medical reason to use MRI.

□□□

32

Echocardiography

Quantitative assessment of myocardial function is of great importance in the diagnosis, treatment, and management of heart diseases and also in the understanding of their physiopathology. It's a non-invasively assess myocardial function. Bidimensional (2D) and M-mode measurements such as systolic left ventricular diameter and index volume or fractional shortening (%FS) are often used as indices of myocardial performance.

Tissue Doppler imaging (TDI) and its derived modalities, strain (St) and strain rate (SR) imaging, are newly-developed ultrasound techniques permitting quantitative assessment of myocardial function by calculating myocardial velocities in real time and by measuring myocardial segmental deformation (contraction or stretching) and rate of deformation

1. The pulsed-wave TDI mode provides information on myocardial movements through a single sample volume, which is placed within the myocardial wall thickness. When the myocardium moves towards the transducer, myocardial velocities are positive (above the baseline). Conversely, when the myocardium moves away from the transducer, myocardial velocities are negative (under the baseline).
2. This color M-mode TDI tracing of the left ventricular free wall (radial motion) shows on the same image both systolic and diastolic velocities within the entire wall thickness. Myocardial velocities towards the transducer are encoded in red, and those away from the transducer in blue. Using a specific software, the mean myocardial velocity (defined as the average of velocity

values measured along each M-mode scan line throughout the myocardial wall thickness) may then be calculated throughout the whole cardiac cycle.

3. Using the 2D color mode, myocardial velocities are superimposed on 2D mode images (here right parasternal transventricular short axis view). Velocities towards the transducer are colored in red whereas those away from the transducer are colored in blue.

Advantages of 2D color TDI mode over the two others

- Ability to simultaneously quantify myocardial velocities in several segments within 1, 2 or 3 walls, thereby allowing assessment of intra- and interventricular myocardial synchrony

Factors of variation: The main factors of variation of TDI variables are:

- Breed,
- Heart rate,
- Anesthesia.

Current applications of the TDI technique

- Offers a non-invasive, sensitive, and quantitative analysis of regional myocardial motion.
- The detection of slight myocardial alterations that are equivocal or even not apparent using conventional ultrasound techniques.
- TDI is more sensitive than conventional echocardiography in detecting preclinical regional myocardial abnormalities before occurrence of left ventricular dilation and over systolic dysfunction.

TDI may also be used to accurately investigate myocardial dysfunction associated with heart diseases, thus providing new insights in the understanding of their pathophysiology. For e.g, diastolic dysfunction has traditionally been thought to be the only abnormality in cats with Hypertrophic Cardio Myopathy (HCM). But using the 2D color TDI mode showed that systolic dysfunction is an additional component of myocardial alteration. Such a systolic dysfunction is characterized by a decrease in longitudinal systolic velocities and gradients (despite normal or increased fractional shortening) and the high prevalence of post-systolic contraction waves.

Two-dimensional speckle tracking echocardiography

2D STE is the most recent ultrasound technique developed in cardiology to assess regional myocardial function concomitantly in several segments

Principle: based on the formation of speckle patterns due to reflection, scattering and interferences between tissue and ultrasound beams in routine gray scale 2D echocardiographic images.

These speckles appear as small, bright elements homogeneously distributed within the myocardium on 2D mode images. They represent natural acoustic tissue markers that can be tracked from frame to frame throughout the cardiac cycle.

Advantages

- Its independence of both cardiac translation and insonation angle.
- Direct measures of myocardial displacement, whereas with Doppler-based techniques, all measurements are done in reference to an external point, *e.g.*, the transducer.

❑❑❑

33

Nuclear Scintigraphy

A highly sensitive imaging technique in which radioisotopes are used to detect functional abnormalities in body systems. A radio pharmaceutical is injected into the blood stream. It gets localized in a particular tissue or organ. Emission of gamma rays from the site can be detected using a gamma camera. Most commonly used radioisotope is Technetium – 99m. Pyrophosphate for bone and for lungs-macro aggregated albumen. It is clinically useful in the diagnosis of functional disorders of kidney, liver, GIT, lungs and thyroid gland. Most commonly used for diagnosis of bone and joint disorders and cancer diagnosis.

Radionuclide used

- Brain – pertechnetate 99m technetium
- Liver – technetium sulphur collide
- Kidney – technetium chelate
- Skeleton – technetium phosphate
- Placenta – labeled human serum albumin
- Lungs – labeled micro sphere

Duration of examination

- Liver and placenta – immediately after injection
- Brain – 1-2 hours after injection
- Kidney – 2 hours
- Abscess/tumor – 48-72 hours

Clinical applications

Most frequently applied clinical examination protocols are described, i.e bone, thyroid, hepatic, renal, brain, cardiac and pulmonary scintigraphy, as well as oncological and inflammation scintigraphy and miscellaneous scintigraphical examinations.

Bone Scintigraphy: seems to be the most frequently performed veterinary nuclear medicine procedure. General injected dose range is 10-20 Megabecquerel(MBq)/body weight in kg. The skeletal scintigraphic examination can be divided into three imaging phases (3-phase bone scintigraphy):

- Vascular phase or blood flow phase or nuclear angiogram (phase I),
- Extracellular or soft tissue phase (phase II),
- Bone phase (phase III).

Major advantage of bone scintigraphy versus radiological examination is that scintigraphy is able to detect abnormalities at a very early stage: a few hours after injury incomplete bone fractures can be detected scintigraphically while radiological abnormalities are detectable only after days

Thyroid Scintigraphy: Thyroid scintigraphy is one of the most common nuclear medicine applications. Recently sodium 99mTechnetium-pertechnetate (99mTcO4-) has been used more extensively for thyroid imaging than radioiodine because of its availability, low cost and radiation safety. Dosage is generally between 37 and 222 MBq for a cat or dog. Intravenously 99mTc-pertechnetate localizes in the thyroid glands 20-30 min after application. Ventral and lateral aspects of the neck region are imagined routinely and additional ventral and lateral views of the neck and thorax should also be acquired to rule out ectopic tissue or tumor metastasis.

Hepatic scintigraphy: There are 3 main forms of hepatic scintigraphy in animals :

- Reticuloendothelial function scintigraphy
- Hepatobiliary scintigraphy
- Portosystemic shunt scintigraphy

Renal Scintigraphy: After intravenous injection of any of the above listed radiopharmaceuticals these will concentrate in the kidneys. Based on localization, mechanism pictures must be taken at different times after administration. Functional renal scintigraphy allows to determine global and individual kidney glomerular filtration rates (GFRs) and effective renal plasma clearance (ERPF).

Brain scintigraphy: Conventional (planar) brain scintigraphy is one of the most simply performable nuclear medicine applications. One to four hours after intravenous application of the radiopharmaceutical static imaging is performed around the head. Dorsal, lateral and caudal images are taken and pictures are evaluated visually. Indications for brain scintigraphy in veterinary medicine differ from human medicine. Suspected intracranial lesions such as tumors, cysts, hemorrhage, abscesses and trauma with head injury are the most frequent indications whereas seizures, cranial nerve disorders, or behavioural changes are much less frequently examined in animals than in humans.

Cardiac scintigraphy: Cardiac scintigraphy contains two main groups of nuclear procedures as

- Myocardial imaging (perfusion and metabolic examinations)
- Functional scintigraphy - is much more frequently performed in the veterinary field.

Pulmonary scintigraphy: Two types of pulmonary scintigraphy methods are known both in human and in veterinary medicine: *ventillation and perfusion examinations*

Oncological and inflammation scintigraphy: All of the listed scintigraphic procedures have the potential chance to detect oncological or inflammation processes in the examined organs but there are especially designed scintigraphical methods for detecting malignancies.

How the procedure works: Nuclear medicine procedures use a radioactive material called a radiopharmaceutical or radiotracer, which is injected into bloodstream, swallowed or inhaled as a gas. This radioactive material accumulates in the organ or area of your body being examined, where it gives off a small amount of energy in the form of gamma rays.

Benefits

- The information provided by nuclear medicine examinations is unique and often unattainable using other imaging procedures.
- For many diseases, nuclear medicine scans yield the most useful information needed to make a diagnosis or to determine appropriate treatment, if any. Nuclear medicine is less expensive and may yield more precise information than exploratory surgery.
- Because the doses of radiotracer administered are small, diagnostic nuclear medicine procedures result in low radiation exposure, acceptable for diagnostic exams. Thus, the radiation risk is very low compared with the potential benefits.

Nuclear medicine diagnostic procedures have been used for more than five decades, and there are no known long-term adverse effects from such low-dose exposure. Allergic reactions to radiopharmaceuticals may occur but are extremely rare and are usually mild. Injection of the radiotracer may cause slight pain and redness which should rapidly resolve.

Nuclear medicine procedures can be time-consuming. It can take hours to days for the radiotracer to accumulate in the part of the body under study and imaging may take up to several hours to perform. The resolution of structures of the body with nuclear medicine may not be as clear as with other imaging techniques, such as CT or MRI. However, nuclear medicine scans are more sensitive than other techniques for a variety of indications, and the functional information gained from nuclear medicine exams is often unobtainable by any other imaging techniques.

❑❑❑

34

Gamma Camera

A gamma camera is a specialized camera encased in metal that is capable of detecting radiation and taking pictures from different angles. It may be suspended over the examination table or it may be beneath the table. Often, gamma cameras are dual-headed with one camera above and one camera beneath the table. The camera could also be located within a large, doughnut-shaped scanner similar in appearance to a computed tomography (CT) scanner

A gamma camera consists of three main parts: A collimator, A detector and Electronic systems.

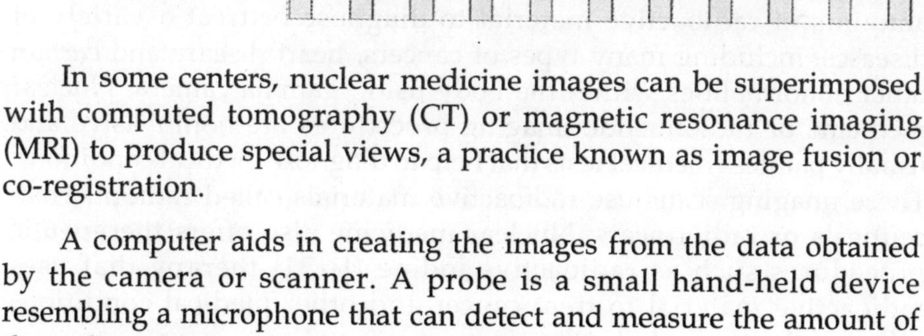

In some centers, nuclear medicine images can be superimposed with computed tomography (CT) or magnetic resonance imaging (MRI) to produce special views, a practice known as image fusion or co-registration.

A computer aids in creating the images from the data obtained by the camera or scanner. A probe is a small hand-held device resembling a microphone that can detect and measure the amount of the radiotracer in a small area of your body.

A positron emission tomography (PET) scanner is a large machine with a round, doughnut shaped hole in the middle, similar to a CT or MRI unit. Within this machine are multiple rings of detectors that record the emission of energy from the radiotracer in your body. A gamma camera, PET scanner, or probe detects this energy and with the help of a computer creates pictures offering details on both the structure and function of organs and tissues in your body.

The radiotracer is either injected into a vein, swallowed or inhaled as a gas and eventually accumulates in the organ or area of your body being examined, where it gives off energy in the form of gamma rays that are detected by gamma camera.

Factors which affect the choice of Tracer

- Gamma rays are chosen since alpha and beta particles would be absorbed by tissues and not be detected outside the body.
- Technitium-99m is most widely used because it has a half-life of 6 hours.
- Unlike other imaging techniques, nuclear medicine imaging studies are less directed toward picturing anatomy and structure, and more concerned with depicting physiologic processes within the body, such as rates of metabolism or levels of various other chemical activity
- Areas of greater intensity, called "hot spots" indicate where large amounts of the radiotracer have accumulated and where there is a high level of chemical activity. Less intense areas, or "cold spots", indicate a smaller concentration of radiotracer and less chemical activity.

Nuclear medicine is a branch of medical imaging that uses small amounts of radioactive material to diagnose or treat a variety of diseases, including many types of cancers, heart disease and certain other abnormalities within the body using gamma camera. Nuclear medicine or radionuclide imaging procedures are noninvasive and usually painless medical tests that help to diagnose medical conditions. These imaging scans use radioactive materials called radiopharmaceuticals or radiotracers. Nuclear medicine also offers therapeutic procedures such as radioactive iodine (I-131) therapy that uses radioactive material to treat cancer and other medical conditions affecting the thyroid gland.

❑❑❑

35

Xeroradiography

Xeroradiography is a type of x-ray in which a picture of the body is recorded on paper rather than on film. It is an alternative method of recording X-ray images, higher in contrast than film-based X-ray imaging. It provides broader latitude and greater edge enhancement than conventional radiography. It is useful in soft tissue imaging such as mammary glands, muscles, tendon and ligaments.

In greek *"xeros"* means "dry"

PRINCIPLE: The production of an image from an X-ray exposure using the charged surface of amorphous selenium, a photoconductor, as the X-ray detector. X-rays passing through objects are received by an X-ray–sensitive metal plate, which is then processed through a unique photocopying-type machine. The recorded image of the object's interior is then transferred onto plastic-coated paper.

Film consists of aluminum plate coated by charged selenium particles. Charged selenium requires light or X-ray to transfer the charge to aluminum plates. On exposure selenium transfers the charge of aluminum plate and become neutral. Negatively charged aerosol spray powder is sprayed on plates and get attached to positively charged selenium. On exposure to light, there is clear cut image formation. The powder picture on the surface of xeroradiographic plate is transferred to a special paper and fixed to form permanent image. It provides enhanced visualization of the borders of different densities (edge effect), low contrast enables differentiation between fat, muscle and bone with exposure latitude and instant picture are available and highly economic. But they cannot be used for very thick parts and requires high radiographic exposure.

In conventional xeroradiography, the image is characterized by a visible edge enhancement, which tends to improve structure visibility over the extent of an image with a wide dynamic range. Because of this ability to show structure detail over a region with wide dynamic range, xeroradiography has found applications in chest radiography as well as mammography and musculoskeletal imaging.

Xeroradiographic imaging process

Step 1

- A uniform charge is deposited on the surface of a highly smoothed selenium plate.
- Xeroradiographic plate consists of a thin sheet of aluminum on which a thin layer of selenium is deposited.
- A very thin aluminum oxide layer is placed as an electric insulator between the selenium and the conducting aluminum plate. The charge is applied by passing the plate in front of a charging scoroton.
- **Scoroton:** A device which creates a corona current for charging selenium plates used in xeroradiography.
- **Corona current:** The ionization current that flows towards a wire maintained at a high potential difference from ground.

Step 2

- The charged plate is placed in a light tight cassette and is exposed to X-rays during the imaging procedure.
- The selenium acts as a photoconductor and the positive charge discharges in proportion to the X-ray flux incident on the selenium plate.
- The distribution of X-ray flux is thus recorded as a distribution of latent positive charge on the selenium surface.

Step 3

- The latent positive charge distribution is developed or made visible by a process which deposits charged toner particles on the selenium plate in proportion to the remaining latent charge on the plate.

- Development is performed using a process known as powder cloud development. In which an aerosol of charged toner particles is created and a back-bias voltage is applied to attract the toner particles of the desired charge to the plate.
- A voltage is also applied to a development electrode placed just in front of the selenium plate which serves to remove non-uniformities from the developed image.
- It is the powder cloud development process that results in the edge enhancement that is characteristic of xeroradiographic images.

Powder cloud development: Attracting either the positively charged or the negatively charged toner particles to the distribution of residual positive electrostatically charged selenium plate, Later the toner distribution is transferred to plastic coated paper.

Toner: Small pigmented dust particles used in the development process of selenium plates in xeroradiography.

Step 4

- The toner on the selenium plate is transferred to a paper sheet and permanently fixed within the plastic coating on the paper.

Step 5

- The plate is cleaned to remove all remaining toner particles and prepared for re-use. Charging is performed only when the plate is ready for use.

Xeroradiography has been used most extensively for mammography applications, Because of the inherent intensity equalization which appeared to allow more uniform detectability. Unfortunately, the dose efficiency for xeroradiography systems is low and for that reason the systems have not achieved high utilization.

Advantages of Xeroradiography

The primary advantage that Xeroradiography imaging offers the prosthetist over that of conventional film radiography (x-ray) is the clarity of the bone's boundary lines. This fact is due to the character of the Xeroradiographic imaging process itself.

Previously, when consulting x-rays of a residual limb, prosthetists either had to accept the blurred contours of the patient's bony anatomy, or were deprived of a lucid image of the soft tissue edges. Instead, each Xeroradiograph can replace two x-ray film pictures (a bone picture and a soft tissue picture) and thus provide the prosthetist with more accurate and easily observable information at a glance.

The Xeroradiograph is developed on opaque paper, usually on a blue format. Unlike x-rays, the Xeroradiograph can be easily stored since there is no need for a viewing box. The rich blue color of the properly exposed negative mode Xeroradiograph serves to enhance the clarity of the image.

Further, the usefulness of Xeroradiography for prosthetics becomes even more obvious when it is pointed out that less magnification takes place in the procedure. More magnification typically occurs on conventional film x-ray because the x-ray cassette is positioned further from the residual limb.

Disadvantages of Xeroradiography

The Xeroradiographic plate is **9 1/2" x** 13 5/8". As a result, it is not possible to photograph a long residual limb in its entirety. Symes level as well as long above knee residual limbs requires two pictures merely to complete the image for one projection. To rectify this problem, the radiology technician must tape a radiographically opaque reference marker onto the midsection of the residual limb prior to imaging. The marker aids the prosthetist in piecing the two pictures together correctly. An alternative to this mosaic approach, of course, is to obtain conventional radiographs of the longer residual limbs.

A second disadvantage of Xeroradiography is that the image is backwards. As a result, when consulting the Xeroradiograph, the prosthetist must recognize that the xeroradiograph is a mirror image of the object. Finally, with Xeroradiography, the patient is usually exposed to a greater radiation dose. The exact difference in radiation exposure between Xeroradiography and x-ray varies, depending on the type of x-ray screen, film, filters, and resulting technique that is used for a comparison.

Generally, using the Xeroradiography technique that we suggest, the local bone Radiation dose appears to be as much as nine times that of conventional x-ray film technique". Although this is undesirable, the amount of radiation both in terms of skin dose, as well as estimated bone marrow dose, is neither alarming nor considered dangerous to the patient, mainly because usually only one Xeroradiograph series is necessary for the animal.

□□□

36

Doppler Imaging

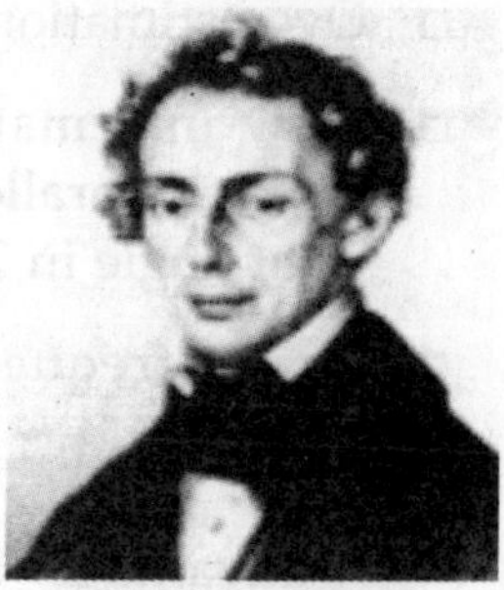
Fig.120 - Johann Christian Andreas Doppler (1803-1853)

Christian Johann Doppler: an Austrian mathematician and scientist first described the physical effect which now bears his name (fig.120). In 1842, he postulated that certain properties of light emitted from stars & presented a paper entitled "On the Coloured Light of double Stars and Some Other Heavenly Bodies." *He suggested the colored appearance of some stars was caused by their motion relative to the earth, the blue (moving toward) and the red (moving away) from earth.*

Principle: An observer stationed on a highway overpass readily notices that the pitch of the sound made from the engine of a passing automobile changes from high to low as the car approaches and then travels into the distance. The engine is emitting the same sound as it passes beneath, but the observer notices a change in pitch dependent upon the speed of the auto and its direction.

Doppler Echocardiography is a noninvasive method. No side effects known, even with frequent and repeat testing. It measures the direction, velocity and disturbance of RBC's moving through the heart & great vessels & differentiates its flow. The technique is used for detection of cardiac valvular insufficiency and stenosis & other abnormal flows in heart. Gives functional information regarding

- ❒ Intracardiac hemodynamics
- ❒ Systolic and diastolic flow

- Blood velocity and volumes
- Severity of valvular lesions
- Location and severity of shunts
- Assessment of diastolic function

Advantage

- Quantitative information regarding pressure gradient across stenotic valves can be achieved.
- Shunting lesions can be documented and quantitated even if they are too small to be seen with 2-D echocardiography.
- Overestimation of blood velocity will not occur.
- Flow information is obtained when the Ultrasound beam is directed parallel to the moving target (i.e. blood flow) instead of right angle in 2-D and M-mode image.
- Lower frequency transducer used, favours recording high velocity.

Disadvantage: Parallel alignment with blood flow is necessary during the interrogation.

Doppler Technique Modalities: There are several modes of doppler echocardiography:

Spectral Doppler: Here the velocity of blood flow is calculated in a region of interest selected by moving a cursor. A graph of blood flow velocity against time is shown, usually with a simultaneous ECG display. Blood flow velocities toward the transducer are displayed as positive (above the baseline), and blood flow velocities away from the transducer are displayed as negative (below the baseline).

The Doppler shift can also be represented by an audible sound, because the shift in frequency is usually quite small and within the audible range (around 10 kHz), so that most machines will show a visual spectral display with a simultaneous audible signal. Spectral Doppler is usually recorded with guidance from two-dimensional echocardiographic images (2D-Doppler, or Duplex Doppler). This allows a cursor to be superimposed over a 2D image, showing the angle of interrogation of the Doppler beam in two dimensions. Spectral

Doppler can be further subdivided into pulsed wave, continuous wave and high-pulse repetition frequency.

1. PULSE WAVE (PW) DOPPLER

The ultrasound waves are transmitted as pulses of waves, with the transducer acting at different times as a receiver or transmitter of ultrasound waves, allowing the interrogation of blood flow velocities within a specific region of interest. This region of interest is represented as a *sample volume on the cursor*. Pulsed wave Doppler has limitations in the maximum velocities that it can display without ambiguity: high velocities result in "aliasing," where blood flow will be displayed as both positive and negative velocities (i.e., signal wraps around the baseline). The velocity at which aliasing will occur depends on the *Nyquist limit (half the pulse repetition* frequency), with higher velocities without aliasing achieved at lower transducer frequencies, and reduced depth from the transducer.

2. CONTINIOUS WAVE (CW) DOPPLER

In contrast, with continuous wave (CW) Doppler, ultrasound waves can be transmitted and received simultaneously. This allows much higher velocities to be displayed, but it is not possible to draw any conclusions about the depth along the cursor from where these velocities are originating (i.e., there is *range ambiguity-* along a specific line).

3. HIGH PULSE REPETATION FREQUENCY (highPRF) DOPPLER

High-Pulse repetition frequency Doppler is a form of pulsed Doppler that shares some similarities with Continuous Wave Doppler. Frequent pulses of ultrasound waves are produced so that a number of sample volumes will be superimposed on the 2D image. This not only allows the display of higher velocities without aliasing, but also increases the number of possible sites from which the velocities are being recorded

Colour Flow (CF) Doppler: In contrast, with continuous wave (CW) Doppler, ultrasound waves can be transmitted and received simultaneously. This allows much higher velocities to be displayed, but it is not possible to draw any conclusions about the depth along the cursor from where these velocities are originating (i.e., there is *range ambiguity-* along a specific line).

Used to record blood flow from a given area comprising numerous sampling points. Color flow system commonly have three types of CF Doppler maps:

- Red (towards inducer)/ blue (away)
- Color: if enhanced (faster blood low)/darker(slower)
- Velocity/variance: shown in green & indicates turbulence or irregular flow (i.e. multiple velocities & direction of blood flow). Here the blood flow is coded in red (toward the transducer) or blue (away from the transducer) and superimposed on the black-and-white 2D image.

Color flow Doppler represents the velocity and direction of blood flow in color, superimposed on a black-and-white 2D image. In effect, the color is displayed within a very large sample volume superimposed on the 2D image. Blood flow away from the transducer is shown in blue, and blood flow toward the transducer is displayed in red ("BART:" blue away, red toward). Disturbed or turbulent flow may be displayed in green or yellow. Aliasing may also occur in color flow Doppler.

Tissue Doppler Imaging (TDI): Here the velocity of myocardial motion is displayed.

More sophisticated machines may include facilities for recording the velocity of myocardial motion. The signals reflected by the moving myocardium are high amplitude, but low velocity. These myocardial velocities can be displayed in spectral format, as a color display, or as color M-mode. It is believed that TDI indices may have advantages over conventional echocardiographic indices, because they may be less influenced by loading conditions.

Power Doppler: similar to color Doppler, uses color to encode blood flow information. But unlike color Doppler, power Doppler information represents the integrated Doppler power spectrum. In other words, power Doppler color encodes based on the amplitude of the turning Doppler frequency shifts. The hue and brightness of the color signal represents the power of the Doppler signal, which is related to the number of moving RBC producing the Doppler shift.

The main advantage of power Doppler is the greater sensitivity to low velocity (i,e low volume) flow because noise has low power and if present, noise in Power Doppler has a uniform background. Power Doppler is also angle independent and no aliasing occurs. The main disadvantages of Power Doppler are the motion or "flash" artifact arising from moving tissue. This artifact has been greatly reduced with new version of power Doppler. Also power Doppler provides no information on flow velocity nor direction.

Power Doppler is useful in situations where there is low velocity and therefore low volume flow in small vessels is expected. Power Doppler is not useful in moving tissue; hence organs moving with respiration (eg. Liver) are difficult to obtain useful Power Doppler images.

□□□